STORIES
THE FEET
CAN TELL

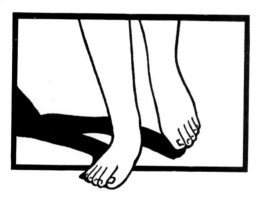

"Stepping to Better Health"

By
EUNICE D. INGHAM
Member N.Y. State Society of Medical Masseurs

PRICE $3.95 SOFT COVER

(Reflexology Color Chart $2.00)

Postage and Handling Each 50¢ Extra

INGHAM PUBLISHINGS
Post Office Box 8412
Rochester, New York 14618

*260,000 copies published
as of January 31, 1975*

How beautiful upon the moun-

tains are the feet of him that

bringeth good tidings.

ISAIAH 52:7

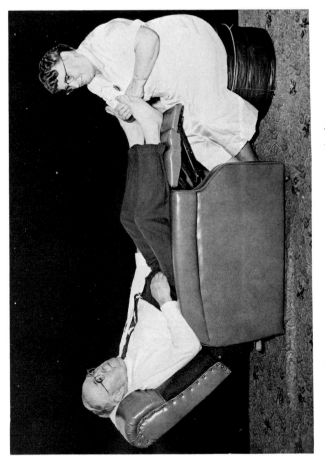

Ideal position for applying reflex technique to the feet.

PREFACE

As author of this little book, I will endeavor to bring to light and explain the actual location of the various reflexes in the feet, as discovered by a careful study in my practice as a masseuse, with hundreds of patients, with whom I have had astonishing results.

Founder of Zone Therapy

Dr. Wm. H. FitzGerald, founder of ZONE THERAPY, held a position that commands respect. He was a graduate of the University of Vermont, and spent two and one-half years in the Boston City Hospital. He was a member of the staff in the Central London Nose and Throat Hospital, and for two years he was in Vienna, where he was assistant to Professor Politzer and Professor Otto Chiari, who are known wherever medical textbooks are read.

While head of the Nose and Throat Department of St. Francis Hospital, Hartford, Conn., his discovery of the Chinese method of ZONE THERAPY was brought to the attention of the medical world, pointing out the fact that pressure, and the massaging of certain zones, has a definite effect in bringing about normal physiological functioning in all parts of the zone treated, no matter how remote this area may be from the part upon which the treatment is exerted.

Dr. FitzGerald, in his work entitled ZONE THER-APY, blazes the path for these further developments as he brings to light for our consideration his discovery of the ten various zones of the body and location of each organ in the body in one or more of these zones.

I want to mention here that I owe a debt of gratitude for my success in this field, to my great teacher, Joe S. Riley, M. D., and his wife, whose names are familiar to many of you as pioneers in the field of ZONE THERAPY.

It was my privilege to be associated with them for several years in their general practice, during which time the methods which will be described in this book, were successfully practiced on hundreds of patients who visited his office.

Each reflex and point of contact has been carefully and thoughtfully checked and rechecked, until with all confidence we call your attention to these findings, sincerely trusting they will prove helpful and beneficial to others.

I hope that these following pages may prove to be another stepping stone to greater heights along this new but effective way of helping those who seek for better health and efficiency.

EUNICE D. INGHAM

INTRODUCTION

The foundation theory of this work as set forth in the following pages has been built up entirely on the opinions of practicing physicians who have had the opportunity of observing the remarkable results obtained from this particular form of compression massage.

So let me say should any one, physician or layman, after a careful study and application of this method, have any valuable suggestions in the form of an explanation to offer, I will be glad to hear from them. Like every new development, it must prove its efficiency to many a doubting skeptic, before being accepted as an established fact.

Many of you will remember, not so long ago, the attitude manifested when the X-ray was first brought to the attention of the world. Yet today it is acknowledged by all a most valuable asset to the success of the medical profession.

We learn from the work of Dr. John C. Hemmeter entitled "Master Minds in Medicine" that it was not until toward the end of the sixteenth century that intellectual Europe was ripe for the acceptance of the discovery of the circulation of the blood. Dr. Michael Servetus planted the seed--Dr. Columbo watered it and to Dr. William Harvey remained the troublesome work of the harvest. And what we possess today in knowledge of the circulation of the blood, we possess through him who, armed only with a magnifying glass, accomplished such great things in spite of bitter criticism.

STORIES THE FEET CAN TELL

I have chosen the unique title, "Stories the Feet Can Tell," for my work because I believe it is possible to learn many a valuable story from the use of this compression massage on the feet. A careful study and application of the methods as described and set forth in the following pages and illustrations, may reveal many a hidden secret of some weakness here or there that may not be manifesting itself yet in any serious degree.

Perhaps a sluggish liver is responsible for the trouble in the intestinal tract that results in constipation. Can the feet be made to tell the story so that the cause of that constipation may be found? Let us see if we find the nerve endings in the right foot reflexing to the liver very tender. If so we know there is a crystal-like formation there interfering with the circulation of the blood to the liver, preventing it from functioning normally. As we massage and work this out we are giving nature a chance to carry away the waste matter and restore the normal circulation to the affected part or parts.

You can readily see how necessary it is that we keep the chemical balance of our blood stream normal and free from crystalline deposits so the feet will have no serious stories to tell. We are all familiar with what the effect of sand or gravel would be in a garden hose, yet we expect our body to function properly regardless of obstructions in the delicate nerve endings.

We forget that our body is supposed to contain about 22 miles of tubing. Every inch of this tubing is kept in activity by contraction and relaxation, dependent entirely upon the muscular activity of the individual. Thus we can see the benefit of any form of massage or exercise that might increase the circulation and strengthen the action of our muscles.

No matter what line of healing you may follow at the present time keep this book at hand, and where others fail to bring about the desired results, try this simple method of producing a reflex action (by manipulation) through the nerve endings on the soles of the feet.

A few case records are given in this book to emphasize the results that have been obtained, which are in no way overdrawn or overestimated. I am enthusiastic only to the extent of the success I have already obtained in my own experience as a masseuse.

And now with the very best wishes for the success of every one who is willing to try it out, I will pass on and explain to the best of my ability, the exact reflex method to be used in the treatment of various ailments.

Don't let the common mistake of its simplicity rob it of any importance. The why and wherefore I am not prepared to explain, I only ask that you try it out. My sincere wish is that every one will become proficient and successful in this great work.

PERFECT HEALTH SPELLS
PERFECT FEET

As soon as we allow the muscles of our body to weaken, the muscle tissue in our feet gives way. The body structure goes down and one or more of the twenty-six bones in each foot may become misplaced causing undue pressure on some nerve ending. This shuts off a certain portion of the normal nerve and blood supply in the bottom of the feet, and as any part of the blood stream becomes choked, it slows down the circulation. As the result of this slowing down of the circulation we have a formation of chemical deposits or waste matter forming in and around the misplaced joints.

While this condition remains in the feet it is diagnosed as broken arches. Let it exist long enough and finally we discover trouble in another part of the body. If this obstruction happens to be in the nerve ending or reflex leading to the kidneys, we find the kidneys are being robbed of a part of their blood supply. This in turn interferes with the proper contraction and relaxation that is necessary in order that the kidneys may carry on their part of eliminating the uric acid from the system. The more of these deposits that have formed, the longer we will have to work with this deep compression massage to dissolve them so that nature can carry away and dispose of this waste matter. This restores the normal circulation to the one or more organs involved.

Again we find another cause for a formation of waste matter or crystal-like formation in the nerve endings where the construction of every bone and muscle of the foot is apparently normal. Perhaps we have inherited or otherwise acquired a certain weakness of some part or organ of the body. The normal muscular activity of that organ is lessened and its function of contraction and relaxing is interfered with. So there has not been sufficient force of circulation to keep that nerve ending free and clear.

A misplaced vertebra, in any part of the spine, will be sure to cut off the normal circulation and interfere with the contracting and relaxing of the part which is depending upon this particular nerve for its blood supply.

Where this may be the cause, we find the corresponding location in the spinal reflexes, as shown in Fig. 5, very tender, but by applying plenty of this compression massage treatment to the reflex leading to this vertebra, we will be sure to help nature repair whatever may have gone haywire. In studying a chart of the nervous system we can see how utterly dependent it is upon the spine for its blood supply; even the slightest undue pressure in any part of the spine cannot help but interfere with the contracting and relaxing process necessary to keep the nerve endings of the feet to that part involved free from any crystalline deposits.

Our body is said to be sixty per-cent fluid. How necessary it is to have this flowing through the tissue in a healthy condition and not over burdened with poisonous acid.

ZONE MARKINGS

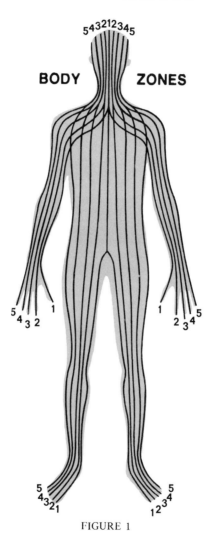

BODY ZONES

FIGURE 1

A study of this diagram will graphically place in the mind the zones of the body.

As there are ten fingers and toes, we may conceive ten zones of the limbs and all parts of the body.

ZONE THERAPY

Now when you proceed with this Chinese method of ZONE THERAPY and begin with the firm pressure of your thumb to examine the reflexes of the feet, you will soon determine the location of the trouble that is sending out the danger signal. Your patients will be amazed that you find such sore places which they had no idea could possibly be found on their feet, since no trouble in the form of any foot discomfort had ever manifested itself in any way to them.

Then again we hear people say, "Oh, my feet hurt, I am sick all over," yet little attention is given by them to see if these pains or disturbances felt at various times might be a warning of a new weakness here or there, not yet manifested in any other part of the body.

A CORN HERE AND CALLOUS THERE

They try one shoe after another, one hurting here and one hurting there. They visit various Podiatrists who are caring scientifically for many minor foot ills to which mankind is heir. Yet their trouble continues, a corn here, a callous there, to impede the natural source of circulation. Yet little do they realize that this undue pressure on some important nerve ending may result in possible injury to each organ dependent upon this particular source for its nerve evergy.

This work being the outcome of my study of

ZONE THERAPY, I have been granted permission by Dr. J. S. Riley to use his chart on Zone Markings for the purpose of giving you an idea of the ten zones of our body and how to locate them.

TEN ZONES

As you will see, we have ten fingers and ten toes, our whole organism being divided into ten zones. From a study of the chart, Fig. 1, you can readily see what we mean by the ten zones of our body. Each line is drawn through the center of its respective zone, and the entire zone includes all parts and organs through which the respective zone line passes.

The right and left sides of the body are the same and each zone passes through the body from front to back, or from back to front. This is true of the legs and arms, also the feet and hands.

LOCATING THE ZONES

Take any of the internal organs of the body, and determine what zone lines pass through them according to the chart. Then picture in your mind on what part of the foot this line will be found and this will guide you somewhat in finding the desired reflex. It is neither hard nor difficult and will only require a little study and practice to make you as proficient as any one in determining the location to be manipulated for any ailment. The fact that it all seems so simple will in no way take away or prevent you from obtaining results. Allow me to say, and emphasize it too, your persistent efforts will be rewarded by many a happy surprise by following the technique found in "Stories The Feet Can Tell."

REACTIONS MANIFESTED

In giving this treatment, you will find that the intensity of the pain will be in direct proportion to the amount and possibly the size of the crystals, and the length of time these crystals have been accumulating. Now as we continue this heavy deep massage, directly over the tender place for a period of five to ten minutes, we are rubbing or grinding, these small sharp needle-like crystals into the muscle tissue and almost invariably the second and third treatment will be even more painful than the first. At each treatment we are causing an acceleration of the circulation of the blood through the affected parts, thus increasing the vitality and endurance of the patient. The irritation set up by these crystals naturally causes a reaction.

VARIATIONS IN REACTIONS

It will be interesting to note the variation of reactions in different patients. Just as no two persons react the same to any condition or circumstance in life, just so will each one have a different reaction although seemingly suffering from the same ailment. For this reason, you must use your own judgment in the length of time given to each treatment, and just how frequently the treatments are to be given. Keep in mind first and uppermost what you are doing. You are stimulating the circulation, and as you stimulate the circulation you raise the body vitality, and as the vitality increases, nature has the strength to overcome and throw off the poisons in the system.

The more of this toxic material the blood contains, the more severe will be the reaction. Many times it manifests itself in the form of a severe cold. This is nature's way of cleaning house and eliminating the poisons from the system. Sometimes this happens after the first treatment, but usually it is the second or third treatment that produces this desired effect. If one has a tendency to respond quickly to any form of treatment, the sooner the reaction takes place, just that much sooner will an improvement in the condition be realized from these treatments. I consider it impossible to fully realize, or to in any way estimate, the amount of good that may be accomplished in various cases by work of this kind.

It is here you must remember the possibility of being too severe. If the patient is nervous and high strung, with extremely sensitive reflexes, you must use only a slight pressure at first. Do not give the treatment too often; never more than twice a week in a case of this type.

REFLEXES PRESENT IN THE HANDS AND FEET

These same reflexes exist in our hands in the same proportion, location, etc., as in our feet. Only it is more difficult to locate them for they are not so pronounced, and the added amount of exercise we give our hands keeps the tenderness worked out, which would otherwise be found.

Our foot we carefully preserve in a shoe, which prevents a certain amount of the natural motion of the foot that would take place if we were constantly walking barefoot in the primitive way nature intended us to follow.

It is estimated that the average pair of feet lift for their owner a total of at least ten cars of coal in weight daily. We forget all this and then wonder why so many people today complain of foot discomfort.

Nature intended that we should walk, bend, twist our feet, and also run occasionally to keep a fresh supply of blood, with the normal circulation surging through every minute joint and nerve extremity of our feet.

But if we allow an excess acid condition to form in our blood stream, we increase the calcium deposits. Then acid crystals, similar to particles of frost when examined under microscope, form in these nerve endings, thus impeding the normal circulation of the blood to the various parts of the body.

CONSTANT MOTION

Our whole body is constantly in motion; the Lungs, Heart, Liver, Kidneys, Intestines, etc. These, when in a perfectly healthy condition, are constantly, day and night, performing their respective duties.

The natural muscular activity of each organ does its part to see that its whole nerve canal is kept free from any detrimental obstruction. But if any one of these members becomes sluggish, weak or injured in any way, it slows down its normal muscular activity to the extent that the extremities of these nerve endings will become clogged. Although only obstructed to a slight degree, yet it may be sufficient to impede the circulation as it returns to supply that organ again with a fresh supply of blood.

It is by the pressure of the thumb coming in contact with these crystals at the nerve endings that causes the pain felt so keenly at these reflexes during the treatment. As they become dissolved by this process of massage, the blood carries them away gradually as it makes its circuit to the feet and back to the heart at the rate of about three times a minute.

Let the massage be given with a slow creeping rotary motion, not using the flat ball of the thumb as much as the corner toward the end. Let the pressure be firm, but at the same time, gently at first and gradually increased with as much as you see the patient is able to endure. The thumb nails must be filed comparatively low. You will often be called upon to prove that it is not your thumb nail causing this pain so keenly felt as you bear down with a firm pressure on these nerve endings where there is a formation of crystalline deposits. Remember, it is important to keep your eye on the expression of your patient. This will tell you the instant your thumb comes in contact with the irritated crystal-filled nerve endings.

LOCATION OF REFLEXES

As you sit facing your patient, who is reclining on a couch or table somewhat higher than the stool or chair you will occupy, place the left foot in your right hand; holding the foot firmly. Then with your left hand between the thumb and first finger, clasp the smallest part of the foot, which will be about midway between the base of the toes and lower part of the heel.

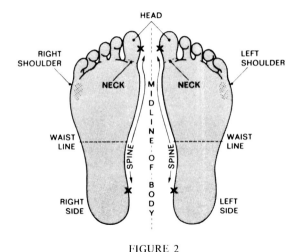

FIGURE 2

This will represent the waist line of the body as shown in Fig. 2. In exact proportion as the organs are located in the body on the left side, above or below this line, the reflex will be found on the sole of the left foot affecting the various parts in the left side of the body. The right foot reflects for the right side in the same proportion. Thus, we find the heart reflected in the left foot, the liver in the right, etc. We have two kidneys, so each foot has a reflex to the kidney on that particular side; the right on the right foot; the left on the left foot.

The ascending colon reflex is on the right foot, as is the right half of the transverse colon, as it traverses the abdomen from right to left just below the liver, stomach and spleen, at about the waist line of the body to the left hypochondriac region on the left side, where it curves downward beneath the lower end of the spleen. Here it is known as the descending colon. This will reflect on the left foot from where it leaves the center of the body.

For instance, a patient with trouble in the colon, or even a lazy colon, will flinch at the slightest pres-

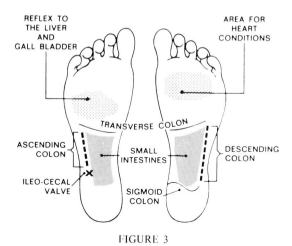

REFLEX TO
THE LIVER
AND
GALL BLADDER

AREA FOR
HEART
CONDITIONS

TRANSVERSE COLON

ASCENDING
COLON

SMALL
INTESTINES

DESCENDING
COLON

ILEO-CECAL
VALVE

SIGMOID
COLON

FIGURE 3

sure at this point of the waist line of the foot. Now to determine if one part of the colon might be affected more than the other, begin with a firm pressure of the left thumb, just above the heel and on the right foot as shown in Fig. 3. Press each portion firmly up the side to the center and across at the waistline of the foot as we have just explained. Then proceed to the other foot and continue the same line of procedure from the inner center line to the side of the left foot and down on the left side following the course of the descending colon in the body.

The point where the greatest amount of tenderness is found will determine the location of the greatest amount of congestion, and where congestion exists disease will result.

THE APPENDIX

You will recall the location of the appendix and how it is situated at the lower border of the ascending colon on the right side. It is a narrow blind-ended worm like tube from three to six inches long and

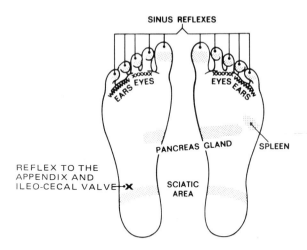

FIGURE 4

held in no set position. Since it is in the right side and below the waist line of the body, just so will you find the reflex to this little organ below the waist line of the right foot, toward the edge, just above the round part of the heel, as shown in Fig. 4.

12

If there is any tendency to a congestion of the appendix, it will show up with a tenderness at this point as you apply a firm pressure with your right thumb. But with a few treatments it can usually be worked out.

I have had marvelous results, in a number of cases, where it seemed almost certain that an operation would be necessary for any relief. One particular case I recall where Mr. P. had already been taken from his work to the hospital for the operation. He finally persuaded the physician to allow him to return home and seek relief with this particular form of compression massage on the reflex of the foot.

The work was carefully directed under the physician's care. When the tenderness in the reflex on the foot had completely disappeared, the discomfort and pain in the region of the appendix had cleared up and to the present time Mr. P. is working every day and feeling fine. (This does not imply that an acute case would not require the attention of a competent physician.)

ILEO-CECAL VALVE

In almost the same location as the appendix we have what is known as the Ileo-cecal Valve. Fig. 4. This forms the opening from the small intestines into the colon, opening toward the large intestine and guarding against reflex from the large into the small bowel. As to whether the appendix or the Ileo-cecal valve is affected will be hard to determine since the location of both is so nearly alike.

Now if the trouble is in that side, and by working out this tenderness we can cause the symptoms to disappear, you need not worry whether it was the appendix or the little valve that was on a strike at the time it was causing the disturbance. If you get results and bring about relief, you are doing all that is expected of you.

When the irritated crystal-filled nerve-endings are massaged, the corresponding organ which if reflexly connected with this particular sensitive nerve receives an added supply of life-giving blood. The congested tissue is thus relieved, and the healing process is hastened.

SMALL INTESTINES

For the small intestines, the reflexes are found above the heel line and below the waist line of each foot. Since the small intestines lie in a part of each of the first, second, third, and fourth zones, we must look for them all the way across from the inside almost to the out-

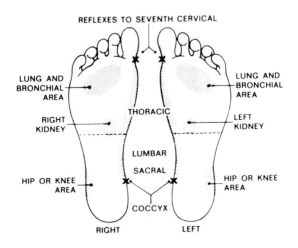

REFLEXES TO SEVENTH CERVICAL

LUNG AND BRONCHIAL AREA

LUNG AND BRONCHIAL AREA

RIGHT KIDNEY

THORACIC

LEFT KIDNEY

LUMBAR

SACRAL

HIP OR KNEE AREA

HIP OR KNEE AREA

COCCYX

RIGHT

LEFT

FIGURE 5

side of the foot, the right half of the intestines showing on the right foot, and the left half on the left foot. Fig. 3.

STOMACH REFLEXES

The stomach is located just a little above the waist line of the body, almost in the center but a little more to the left side. We find its reflex above the waist line of the foot in the first, second and third zones on the right foot, and the first, second, third and fourth zones of the left foot.

LUNGS AND BRONCHIAL TUBES

The lungs and bronchial tubes being on each side alike will be found in the same location on each foot, a little way below the base of the toes. Fig. 5.

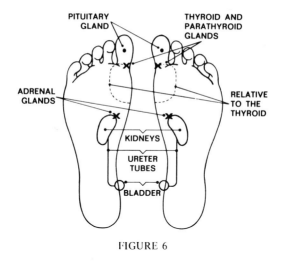

FIGURE 6

PNEUMONIA

Keep this in mind if you are called upon to render relief in case of pneumonia, also the position pictured in Fig. 21. Compression massage at this point will relieve a certain amount of tension which is always helpful in pneumonia. In an acute case let no other reflex be worked without the physician's advice.

GALL BLADDER

This being imbedded in the liver, just off center on the right side, you will find its reflex on the right foot deep in, a little under the ball of the foot as shown in Fig. 3.

KIDNEYS

Each kidney will be reflexed in the second and third zone of each foot, at about the waist line of the foot. Fig. 6.

EYES AND EARS

Location and position for reaching the reflex to the eyes given in Fig. 4 and Fig. 7 reaching down from the top onto the foot at the base of the toes.

BLADDER

Location given in Fig. 6 and Fig. 27. Since the bladder is located in the center of the body we will find the reflex in the first zone on the inside of each ankle.

THE SPLEEN

Shape and Location

The Spleen is a soft, brittle, very vascular, oblong, flattened organ embracing the fundus of the stomach, to which it is attached by the gastro-splenic omentum. This completely invests the spleen except at the helium, and where the suspensory ligament is attached.

Its external surface is convex, smooth, and in contact with the under surface of the diaphragm which separates it from the ninth, tenth, and eleventh ribs of the left side. In size and weight it is liable to extreme variations at different periods of life. In the adult it is usually about five inches in length, three or four inches in breadth, and an inch and a half in thickness, and weighs about seven ounces.

SPLEEN AND THE ZONES

Where Located

This description gives you an idea of the zones in which the spleen is located, so you will have no trouble in locating the reflex in the left foot. Remember its location in regard to the waist line of the body and how it will compare to that of the waist line of the foot, and you will be able to readily place your thumb on the nerve reflex to the spleen. See Fig. 4.

I will not say that you can always determine if this tenderness may mean trouble only in the spleen, for we have other important points of contact so close to that of the spleen.

Lying almost in front of the spleen is the splenic flexure, where the transverse colon passes just in front and below the spleen at the left hypochondriac region where it makes its curve downward beneath the lower end of the spleen. Trouble in this particular part of the colon is very often the case.

SPLEEN OR COLON

Which is Wrong?

But if the patient is inclined to be anemic and has already been diagnosed as such by a physician, and you find a tenderness at this point, you can be sure it is the spleen and not the colon that is in need of your attention. It is possible that both conditions might exist, but one thing is certain, you will be able to remedy the trouble, whatever is wrong, by removing those acid crystals from the nerve endings and supplying the parts with the normal circulation.

REPLACING OLD CELLS WITH NEW

Should the trouble be pernicious anemia, it will take longer to obtain results, so do not be too impatient. It takes time to completely replace new cells in any organ of our body. Therefore, we must wait till nature has exchanged the old for a new model machine before we can look for perfect performance. Do not expect a "model T Ford" to compete with a new Cadillac.

ANEMIC CONDITIONS

I cannot recall a single case of simple anemia where this particular point was not extremely tender, for it is the spleen that manufactures the red blood cells. If this spleen fails to do its work through any means of congestion cutting down its blood supply, in turn it will fail to reproduce the substantial red blood cells necessary for our well-being. The spleen is also the burying ground of the old broken down blood cells which by the laws of nature rise again. They are buried and yet they are manufactured there. Nature takes the old and converts them into the new red blood cells.

DIET BENEFICIAL

It is well to remember that a blood building diet is extremely important in overcoming anemic conditions, let this be directed by a competent nutritionist and combined with this form of compression massage and your efforts will be rewarded with remarkable results.

EYES

We find a big majority of individuals today whose eyesight is affected in one way or another, perhaps nothing more than astigmatism, a slight flattening of the eyeball, or some condition that could be easily corrected by the wearing of glasses.

SOME CASES INCURABLE

Again we have the poor unfortunate souls who have inherited some form of an infection that can never be wiped out. We do not profess to say that any of these can be benefited by this or any other method, but we do find that some conditions can be greatly improved, even to a form of glaucoma, which is a condition where the eyeballs become very hard. It is produced by the fluids forming in quantities beyond the normal, and thus extending the coats of the eye until excessive strain and hardness are felt, with partial or total blindness.

CASE RECORD

Successful With Glaucoma

One particular case I had of this type was seemingly, to all appearance and according to the doctor's diagnosis, cleared up entirely.

Mr. S., a man about 45 years of age, had become extremely discouraged when informed by several specialists that it would be only a matter of time till his sight would be entirely gone. He was advised not to read or tax his eyes in any way unnecessarily in order to prolong the sight he now had.

By examining his feet I found no tenderness at any point except at the reflex to the eyes, which is found between the second and third toe at the point where they are joined to the foot, and a little below, reaching down, as we might say, from the top of the toes as shown in **Fig. 7 & Fig 4.**

We will consider you are working on the left foot, and always have the patient facing you. Now grasp the outside of the foot with your right hand, place your thumb on the sole of the foot, bracing it from the top with your fingers, and with your right thumb reach down from the root of the toes on to the foot in a way to reach the reflex deep down be-

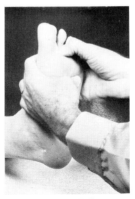

FIGURE 7
Best Position for Reaching the Reflex to
the Eyes and Ears.

tween and around the base of the second and third toes. It may be necessary to use your finger on the right hand to find the exact location. At least don't give up till you have most thoroughly tried with both hands. It may be necessary for you to reverse the procedure outlined, holding the foot in your right hand and using the thumb and first finger of your left hand for this massaging.

This method of massage was carried on persistently, every day, in the case of glaucoma with Mr. S. just mentioned. I was able to see him but once a week, as he lived in a distant city, so I carefully instructed Mrs. S. to follow my direction faithfully by massaging this reflex every day.

After a while Mr. S. called on his specialist, who said he had never known a case to have so greatly improved from the use of the drops he had given him to simply relieve the condition.

Again, later, another visit was made to the same specialist, who said he had never yet seen a case so completely cleared up from the use of these drops. The fact was, Mr. S. had not been using the drops at all since this compression massage had been given to him.

Not caring to hurt the feelings of this specialist, nothing more was said, but Mr. S. was advised now by him to discontinue the use of the drops since the glaucoma had apparently disappeared.

EYES AND THEIR BLOOD SUPPLY

Remember this, where there is any trouble with the eyes caused by some bodily ailment, and you find the place between the toes very tender, it is certain you can help the condition by removing the crystals and replacing the normal circulation.

A tenderness at this point, as in any other place, means the eyes are being deprived of the proper blood supply, which means health and activity to any part of the body. You will notice rapid results from these treatments where there is a burning or itching condition of the eyes.

21

EARS

Now we find the ears too can be greatly benefited, but we will not try to tell you that all forms of deafness will respond to this treatment.

Deafness like blindness, can be caused by various conditions that may render it beyond all human power to restore. But from our past experience, we repeat again how this method has helped hundreds to a better degree of hearing.

Follow carefully the directions given for treating the the eyes. The procedure is practically the same as far as the position for holding and grasping the foot is concerned. Only the reflex for the ears will be found between the third and fourth toes, while for the eyes we work principally between the second and third toes.

For the ears try also between the fourth and fifth toes, in other words hunt till you find a sore place. It is not advisable to follow any concrete rule as to locating these reflexes. It is impossible to tell in just what zone the trouble is that causes the deafness. With some it is one thing, and another something else entirely.

SURPRISING RESULTS OBTAINABLE

I shall not try to overestimate the amount of good that may be accomplished by this treatment, but I will say that you too, like myself, will be surprised many times at the astonishing results you will obtain where you might be expecting them the least. Especially if the deafness happens to be that which is caused by a catarrhal condition which is often the cause.

ENLARGED TONSILS OR
SORE THROAT

Now here comes a patient to you for help with a sore throat or enlarged tonsils. Where will you expect, on the foot, to find the reflex to the throat?

Since it is in the fleshy part of the big toe where we find the reflex to troubles in the head, naturally we will expect to find the throat reflexed at what we call the base of the big toe just at or a little above where it joins on to the foot as shown in Fig. 8.

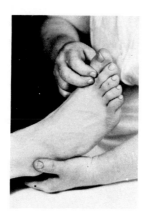

FIGURE 8

Position for Massaging the Reflex to the
Throat.

Let me ask that you think a moment and picture in your mind that the throat is that part which connects the head to the body. Then just so will we find the tenderness reflecting to the throat in that part of the toe where it is connected to the foot. It will be necessary to use the first finger for the greater part of the work of this reflex, as you will have to reach around over the top of the toe on to that side between and facing the second toe. It will only require a little pressure here, not more than can be easily given with the first finger. The thumb may be used for working on the underside of this big toe.

Remember one thing, that the location of the tenderness around this big toe where you will work will depend on just what part or parts of the throat are mostly congested.

POSITION FOR REACHING THE REFLEX TO THE THROAT

If the trouble or congestion in the throat is caused by an excessive amount of poison in the system, you may not get results till that condition has been cleared up, but if this congestion is not of too long standing as the result of a recent cold or sore throat, you will be surprised at what nature will do when she is given the proper amount and quality of blood with which to do her repair work.

You will be surprised how readily a stiff lame neck will loosen up under this form of compression massage around the big toe.

I have had a number of cases where it would seem as if the stiffness simply melted away and where they had come into the office not able to turn the head scarcely at all, they would go out almost as well as ever.

SINUS TROUBLE

This most annoying pain and trouble in the head is very perplexing to both the patient and the practitioner. It is claimed by some to be what was at one time known as catarrh of the head.

TEMPORARY RELIEF

The various forms of local treatment can afford some relief, but it is only temporary. They relieve the effect without doing anything to remove the cause.

Congestion, the keynote to all our aches and pains, whether it be a headache or a toeache, is the cause of our sinus trouble. If it is hard for you to believe it, try it out with this method and see for yourself if what I am telling you is true or not.

TENDERNESS IN TOES

Since this sinus trouble is in the head, we will find the reflex to this in the ten TOES. Where the congestion is severe and of long standing, it will be interesting to note the tenderness that will be found in, on, and around the toes. This will be observed especially as you press toward the base or root of each toe as shown in Fig. 4 and Fig. 9, from the outer and inner side on the ball of all ten toes.

The sides too, will be especially sensitive, and as you persistently continue this procedure, watch the results. The improvement will not be in a minute or over night. It will take time, the duration of which will depend entirely on the vitality and susceptibility to respond, and the length of time the condition has existed.

THE CAUSE AND EFFECT

If this sinus trouble is caused from a catarrhal condition in the system, the result of nature striving to overcome a hyperacidity in the body, we will do well to first try and remedy this condition; the cause of which you may have already found from the discovery of some tender reflex indicating what part or parts may be at fault.

NATURE DOES HER PART

Nature is constantly struggling to eliminate the waste matter of our body. The dead worn out body cells that are being constantly replaced by new ones, must be eliminated from our system in various ways.

One important avenue of escape for these poisons of the system is the pores of our skin. The mucous membrane in the head, nose, and sinus portion, being so much thinner at that particular place, gives nature a chance to discharge her surplus supply more easily through that channel. The result is, we have a discharge from the nose as nature succeeds in throwing it off. If instead, it becomes congested in the head, as in most cases of Sinus trouble that have been known, then the trouble is more serious and painful, and you will wait longer for results.

But do not get discouraged, for as long as the slightest tenderness remain, you are still fighting with congestion.

Now where a condition of sinus trouble continues to exist, we know nature is still overburdened with this toxic acid mucous-forming condition and seeking constantly a form of elimination along the line of least resistance where the membrane lining is the thinnest.

EFFECTS OF A COLD

When you are overtaken by what is commonly known as a cold, remember this is nature's way of eliminating the toxic acid of the system. As a result we have an excessive amount of discharge from the nose and throat; because it is here where this acid can find its exit in the way of least resistance.

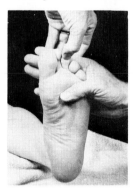

FIGURE 9
Position for Massaging the Reflexes to the
Sinuses.

The old method of soaking the feet in hot mustard water, taking a hot sweat bath, etc., all had its effect in relaxing and opening the pores of the body, helping nature in its process of elimination.

A PHYSICIAN'S METHOD

Our physician with his various remedies today for a cold, endeavors to bring about this same eliminating effect through the use of drugs as a more modern discovery. When people have completely recovered from a cold, note how much better they usually feel for the time being from this house-cleaning method.

HAY FEVER

As late summer approaches you will often be asked if you can do anything to relieve or benefit a condition of hay fever with this form of compression massage on the feet.

Without the slightest doubt, the same method we have just outlined for relief in cases of sinus trouble will also relieve one suffering from hay fever. In fact, I may safely say you will be surprised how quickly results will follow if you persistently work out all the tenderness you can find in, on and around all ten toes.

GLANDS

We find so many today suffering from various ailments, where the original cause can be traced to a gland deficiency. Remember every thought and emotion affects our glands and every thought is either constructive or destructive. Our glands are health builders, each pouring out secretions, which if in harmony, health is the result. If any one of the seven principal glands of the body fail to function, our whole mechanism is out of order.

How necessary then that we remember the importance of right thinking. If we are filled with thoughts of fear, worry, anxiety, or grief, let us shift our mental gears and replace them with those of hope, cheer, courage and happiness. We must do it if we want to be one hundred per-cent well. If mentally depressed, try to associate with those who are optimistic, who are looking on the bright side of life. To be among those who have courage will help us to be more courageous and magnetic physically and mentally.

Our success in life depends on our ability to radiate a pleasing personality, which is wholly dependent on our thoughts and emotions and, how our glands are functioning, if in harmony or out of harmony.

We will now proceed to discuss the various forms of work allotted to the most important members of the gland family. We will first consider the thyroid, and relate a few of the strange pranks for which this gland can be held responsible.

THE THYROID GLAND

When the Thyroid gland refuses to work, the baby no longer grows, but develops a vacant idiotic look. This gland acts somewhat as a spark generator and storage battery for the body. If we let our battery run down we get tired and gain weight rapidly, but if it becomes over charged the Thyroid secretion is excessive, the patient will be nervous, irritable, will lose weight and become emotionally unbalanced. Many times we find this condition responsible for our neurasthenics. It may be advisable to have a metabolism test taken to check up on the activity of this gland, but it has been proven that whatever the case may be, whether we must

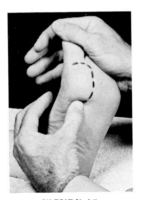

FIGURE 10

Position for Massaging the Reflex Relative
to the Thyroid Gland.

speed up or slow down the activity of this very important gland, we can usually bring about normal balance by this reflex method consisting of this heavy deep massage over the reflex on the foot leading to the Thyroid gland. Fig. 6. This will be found principally in the first and second zone on each foot at the base of the big toe, deeply seated, and must be reached by using the outside corner of the thumb as shown in Fig. 10.

In cases where there is a congestion leading away from the Thyroid toward the ear you will find it tender as you proceed with a deep pressure up between the first and second zones, between the big toe and the second toe. You will notice remarkable results from your work on this reflex. We have known them to gain as much as a pound a week where the gland was overactive and their weight far below normal.

EXOPHTHALMIC GOITRE

In this condition of goitre, the Thyroid gland enlarges, as in the case of simple goitre; the heart beat increases rapidly; the eyes bulge forward; the body becomes emaciated and very weak, and a nervous condition ensues. The growth itself may be scarcely noticeable, yet capable of doing a lot of mischief. Thus to work on the reflex to the Thyroid gland would help a condition of exophthalmic goitre.

We often find this condition has been brought about by a depressed mental attitude, grief or disappointment. No doubt you too, like myself, can recall many a case of this type which had its origin entirely around a thwarted love affair where a depressed desire had a definite effect on this particular gland interfering with its normal functioning.

It may take you longer to correct a case of this type unless you are successful in some way in changing the mental attitude or convincing the patient that to redirect the attention along some constructive line of endeavor is necessary for complete recovery.

THE PITUITARY GLAND

Some term the pituitary as the master gland, for it has a powerful influence over the rhythm of the heart, beating time for the Adrenal and Thyroid glands in maintaining energy for the whole body. The Pituitary gland discharges certain hormones directly into the blood stream, playing an important part in our mode of living. It regulates our growth and governs, to a certain degree, the formation of sugar in our system.

A superactive pituitary gland is responsible for the growth of our giants, while an inactive pituitary is the cause of our dwarfs. If it goes haywire there is no telling what type of monstrosity may be produced.

Prof. Borgas, a surgeon of Rastov, Russia, capitalized in a dramatic way, on the growth-giving power of the pituitary gland. From the brain of a young man, who an hour before had been killed in an automobile accident, Dr. Borgas cut out the pituitary and grafted it into the stunted body of a fifteen year old girl, three feet tall. In six months she grew six inches.

Dr. James Hatton has had good results in reducing high blood pressure with carefully timed X-ray exposure to the back of the patient's head, and the kidneys, over the Pituitary and adrenal regions.

If good results can be obtained by X-ray, then we know good results can be had by any method that will increase the circulation to that particular area. Suppose, as the result of congestion, this gland enlarges and becomes too big for the niche in which it rests, then a headache might follow. Not that all headaches are the result of an abnormal pituitary, but this gland can do a lot of mischief.

A "STORY THE FEET DID TELL"

It may be interesting here to relate an experience I had one day last summer with an ex-champion wrestler who accompanied his wife to my office. Mr. G., with an exaggerated air of skepticism, stood by critically questioning Mrs. G. as to the necessity of her flinching as I massaged the extremely tender reflexes of her feet. I endeavored to explain the cause of the tenderness at the nerve endings. Mr. G. confidently assured me I would find no tender place in his feet, saying, "I would like to meet the person who could make me flinch."

Since his appearance was that of one in perfect health I had no idea that we would be able to demonstrate to him the feeling of a tender reflex. After completing the massage on Mrs. G., she insisted that he should let me try the various reflexes of his feet. As I proceeded, I found no tenderness whatsoever until I reached that of the Pituitary gland as shown in Fig. 6 and Fig. 11. At this point he did not stop to flinch but nearly jumped off the table and cried out in no uncertain tones, that "it did hurt." To prove my findings I made sure the same tender spot existed in the center of each big toe and then I ventured to ask him if he had ever suffered from headaches.

In answering me he said it was impossible to describe the amount of suffering of the severity of the extreme headaches he had endured. It was almost unbelievable the amount of aspirin he had taken. And now comes the most unbelievable part of the story. After his third visit to my office this tenderness had completely worked out. While this took place almost a year ago he has had no return of his headaches. To verify this statement, I called on Mr.

and Mrs. G. about a week ago. If any one feels inclined to doubt the truthfulness of this experience, their name and address will be cheerfully given.

As I have said before, if you will sincerely try out this form of compression massage as directed in this book, you will affirm without fear of successful contradiction that congestion in the head as in any other part can often be relieved by this method of work on certain parts of the feet.

CONGESTION

The Pituitary is one of the smallest glands, being only the size of a pea and weighs about one-sixtieth of an ounce, and is situated in front of the medulla oblongata in the pituitary fossa of the sphenoidal bone.

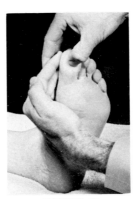

FIGURE 11

Position for Massaging the Reflex to the
Pituitary Gland.

It has much to do with muscular strength and its removal would cause death. Its secretions are entirely internal, and are naturally taken into the system by absorption. Any means of stimulation to this gland, if properly given, will produce strength and health. I know of no better means of stimulating this gland than by this reflex method of ZONE THERAPY that we shall herein outline for your consideration. Note carefully the exact location as indicated in Fig. 6 and Fig. 11.

Since this gland is found resting in a groove at the base of the brain in a bony cradle just above the nasal cavity, we will find our reflex to this in the center of the big toe. You will invariably find this point tender, in cases of any glandular trouble, especially where there is a diabetic condition. It may be somewhat hard to find at first, but persistent pressure with the side of the thumb will be sure to locate it, and a few minutes attention given to massaging for this gland at each treatment will often produce amazing results.

CASE RECORD

If anyone is inclined to doubt the effect that can be produced by a heavy deep massage of the center of the big toe (the Pituitary reflex), read a case I here relate.

Mr. H., 63 years of age, had suffered with intense headaches for over five years dating back to a most serious operation when a brain tumor was removed. It was diagnosed as a cancerous type, and no hope was held out for his life, either during or after the operation. Beyond all expectation he survived and was able to be up and around his peaceful little home in the country, but never with any degree of comfort for he was annoyed with a constant headache during every waking hour, day or night. It was hard to even picture help for such a severe case caused by a most critical operation of this type.

The growth having been mostly on the right side of the head, led me to believe I would find the reflex to that part on the left foot, since certain nerve reflexes cross at the back of the neck. As I proceeded gently around the top of the big toe, on each side, etc., the tenderness was extreme. I continued this massaging for about ten minutes, watching his expression intently so as to determine how deep and what pressure might be used without causing too much discomfort. I knew this tenderness was the result of congestion which must be released before there would be any degree of relief. Then, too, a condition of that kind would mean congestion possibly of the neck and shoulder on that side. So I proceeded to the reflex of the shoulder as shown in Fig. 2 and Fig. 20 and found this too, as tender as the

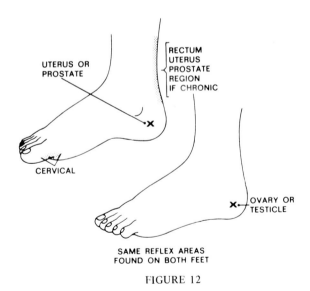

SAME REFLEX AREAS
FOUND ON BOTH FEET

FIGURE 12

reflex to the head. A little persistent work here at the base of the little toe, resulted in some immediate relief. After the third treatment Mr. H. turned to his wife and with tears of joy in his eyes exclaimed, "Mina, for the first time in five years, my headache is gone." The following summer found him again working in his garden.

Another source of annoyance which added greatly to his discomfort, was that of an enlarged prostate gland, which not only increased his nervousness, but disturbed his rest at night by his being aroused six to eight times each night to urinate.

This meant work on the reflex to the prostate gland, which will be found midway between the ankle bone and edge of the heel as shown in Fig. 12.

With the heel of the left foot resting in the palm of your left hand, grasp the ankle with your right hand and try to locate this reflex with a firm rotary motion with the second and third fingers. Steadying your hand from the opposite side with the thumb and natural grasp of the ankle, allowing a free motion of the fingers for the massage, work on and around this particular part. It may take a few moments to locate the tender reflex, but remember where there is any abnormal condition of this gland there will be congestion with a formation of crystals at the nerve ending. This is what you are seeking to find and what you are going to break up, scattering the congestion and replacing the free normal circulation so nature can repair the sick, afflicted part. All she asks of us is to give her a chance.

Just as a person improperly fed and starving for the necessities of life would be incapable of working proficiently, so it is with any portion of our body. If we cut off any part of the circulation with calcium or crystalline deposits, we deplete the functioning of those particular glands and their associate members.

THE PANCREAS

The Pancreas is a compound racemose gland of pyramidal shape about six to eight inches long, one and a half inches wide and one inch thick. It is situated transversely across the posterior wall of the abdomen, behind the stomach and in front of the second lumbar vertebra.

The Pancreatic duct extends the whole length of the gland and opens into the descending part of the duodenum to the inner side, with the common bile duct. As a ductless gland this capable organ secretes from its insular cells, insulin, which acts as a draft to a furnace in burning up the excessive sugar in the system.

While the liver and pancreas secrete differently, the secretions of both are affected in diabetes. It is the function of the pancreas to secrete pancreatic juice and also a fluid of great digestive power known as insulin which burns up or consumes any excessive sugar that might be in the blood stream as the result of a torpid liver.

It is the work of the liver to secrete bile, but if it fails to do this normally, abnormal secretions take place and an oversupply of sugar is manufactured in the liver. Then in the face of this if we find a depleted pancreas unable to send out this important insulin, as a draft to the furnace in burning it up, the blood stream becomes overloaded with sugar and that spills over into the urine, and overburdens the kidneys, too, in throwing it off.

DIABETES

What you are interested in now will be to know if anything can be done to help this pancreas, since it is failing to perform its duty as shown by the presence of sugar in the urine. You will be sure to find its reflex tender, indicating the presence of crystals in the nerve endings. Then as you proceed with this heavy deep massage on the reflex according to the location

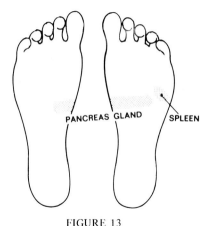

PANCREAS GLAND   SPLEEN

FIGURE 13

outlined in Fig. 13, you will be breaking up these deposits, supplying this gland with a better blood supply which will in time wake it up to a better performance of its duty.

I have had astonishing results from this ZONE THERAPY work in cases of Diabetes but it takes time and patience.

As in every ailment, we find some who respond more readily than others; so do not get discouraged. It has completely cleared up the condition for many.

INSULIN NOT A CURE

If the urine is being tested carefully during this time, it will be interesting to note the increase of sugar showing in the tests the day following your work on this reflex. The increase in circulation evidently stimulates the liver to throw off more of its excessive load of sugar.

If insulin is being used, by all means keep it up until the tests improve sufficiently to warrant, a gradual decrease. If under the care of a physician, he will order the amount to be cut down as the tests improve, for he will be as anxious as you are to see the units of insulin decreased. Insulin is not a cure, but acts only as a crutch to bolster up and supply that which is deficient in the system. The same as if you have a broken limb, the crutch is needed only until that which has been injured is again able to perform its duty.

ASTHMA AND THE ADRENAL GLANDS

Asthma, we all know, is a very disagreeable ailment. It is not considered particularly dangerous, but it can cause a lot of discomfort, and may continue with a devastating effect on the system over a period of years and almost a lifetime in some extreme cases. It is considered a condition where the phlegm hardens in the bronchial tubes.

Since the cause seems to vary in different individuals, it is impossible to expect relief in every case from any one method or form of treatment. We all know that extreme attacks are usually relieved by the use of adrenalin either by hypodermic injection or inhalation of the spray. Would it not seem possible then if we could increase the supply of adrenalin in the system, we might in most cases bring about relief?

LOCATION OF THE ADRENAL GLANDS

We will first call to mind the location of these very important glands, as they sit like little caps one atop each kidney, so closely connected with and related to the kidneys that it would be impossible to determine a difference between the reflex to the kidneys and that of the adrenal glands.

Nevertheless let us remember that we cannot stimulate circulation to one without helping the other; and since it is so important to one suffering from asthma to have a sufficient supply of adrenalin secretion, let us concentrate on doing all in our power to stimulate a better action on these important glands.

NOTHING MORE PRECIOUS

There is nothing more precious to the well-being of an individual than a good pair of adrenal glands. It is the adrenalin secretion that stimulates the action of the heart.

The emotion of fear plays an important part on these adrenalin secretions. Strength is hidden within these glands, which is brought into effect in times of immediate danger. It is the secretion from a good pair of adrenal glands that gives us courage and strength to successfully cope with any emergency in life. The strength and success of our great athletes and prize fighters all depend on the condition and activity of their adrenal glands.

The same important secretion governs the amount of vitality and resistance built up in our body to fight and resist disease. Then allow me to say we can make no mistake in doing anything that will increase the circulation and stimulate the secretions of such an important pair of glands.

I have never yet found a case of asthma where the reflexes to these glands were not tender. Asthma, like any other malady, will not be found in a perfectly healthy body where every gland and organ is functioning in perfect harmony. Thus, many a case of asthma will respond readily to this method when used on the reflex to the adrenal glands. Fig. 6. It may take quite a while in some cases where the difficulty has existed for many years. But time and a little persistent effort on your part will conquer many a seeming impossibility.

DO NERVES AFFECT SKIN ACTION?

It is allotted to our skin to throw off and send out three pints of poison a day. It is said if this were to be injected back into the blood stream we would die in three days of blood poisoning.

Now suppose we are all tightened up worrying over something that tenses and tightens all the pores of the body so that we fail to throw off this allotted portion of poison. We are then increasing the burden of the kidneys and heart which have so much to do with the elimination of the poisons of the body.

ECZEMA

This I give you here as a thought to remember in any case of skin eruption, especially eczema. First see if the kidney action is interfered with by a formation of crystalline deposits in the nerve endings--see if they might be in this way hindered in doing their important part of eliminating the uric acid from the system, thus placing an extra burden on the pores of the skin.

THE HEART

A GREAT PUMPING STATION

Our heart, our blood and its circulation, are most important factors of our being. It is said that 156 pounds per hour of this precious life giving fluid pass through this great pumping station called the heart, on its round to supply the body with nourishing material.

In the Dresden Hygiene Exposition it was shown that 24 quarts of blood pass through the circulatory system in three minutes. In twenty-four hours the heart does enough work to lift three men to the top of a building 44 feet high. Is it any wonder this great organ would grow weary at times?

SIZE, WEIGHT, ETC.

The heart is a hollow muscular organ of a conical form, placed between the lungs and enclosed in the cavity of the pericardium, obliquely in the chest. The broad attached end or base, is directed upwards to the right and corresponds to the interval between the fifth and eighth dorsal vertebrae. The apex is directed forwards and to the left and corresponds to the interspace between the cartilages of the fifth and sixth ribs.

The heart in an adult measures about five inches in length, three and a half inches in breadth, and two and a half inches in thickness. The prevalent weight in the male varies from ten to twelve ounces in proportion to the size of the body.

LOCATING THE REFLEX TO THE HEART

We find the heart and the muscles surrounding it and governing its activity will be reflexed strongly in the left foot and principally in the second, third and fourth zones. Its being embedded deep in the body will necessitate considerable pressure in some cases.

Now with the heel of the left foot resting on the palm of your left hand, use your right thumb; try to locate the reflex at the base of the third and fourth toes as shown in Fig. 14 and Fig. 3.

I suggest you use the inside corner of the thumb for this. It may require a little time and considerable pressure to find the reflex not knowing the exact location of the trouble, whether it be with or around

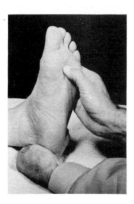

FIGURE 14

Position for Massaging the Reflex to the Heart.

the heart. But any tenderness will be evidence of congestion, and you will have no difficulty in convincing the patient that something is not quite normal, as evident from the tenderness discovered by your pressure on the reflex.

EFFECTS OF CONGESTION

If the slightest congestion takes place among the arteries and veins surrounding the heart and this condition remains long enough, what usually happens-- why, we soon hear of heart attacks.

CONGESTION FORMS CLOTS

Congestion forms clots, and these disturb the vascular action of the heart, called embolus (blood clot in the blood vessels). To call a condition of this kind, "heart disease," is a misnomer. It is like blaming the engine for the poor performance of our automobile, when actually the trouble is caused by an obstruction in the gasoline line robbing it of the necessary amount of gas needed for the proper functioning of the motor.

Palpitation may be caused solely from indigestion. As the stomach, filling with gases formed from undigested food, distends and presses against the diaphragm, it appears to disturb the heart.

AS COMPARED TO A WATCH

Remember the network of muscles constituting the heart and the various valves and intricate parts that go to make up this most important organ. When studying the anatomy of the heart, it always reminds me of a watch, with so many wheels and parts to get out of order.

By this time we can readily understand how undue nerve tension, congestion, etc., in and around the heart, would tend to slow up the action, and finally cause it to stop. Like dust in the delicate wheels of a watch, only sometimes we can restore a watch to action by flushing it with some form of fluid.

But the heart can never be restored when once it has ceased to beat. It is before it stops that it must be flushed with the proper blood supply, which you will be able to give it by freeing these nerve endings of all acid or calcium deposits where there is a tender reflex. Suppose you find no tenderness in this region; then you know the trouble must be something other than of the heart itself. In many cases of heart trouble, results may follow quickly, for so many times, as we have explained, you will find what has been mistaken for heart trouble is only some nerve tension or some tightened muscle, which, when relaxed, will restore the heart again to its normal action.

Let me suggest that your work for the heart be given rather easy at first. When you find the tender place, work on it for two or three contacts, then let that place rest, while you work some other parts, then return to it again. Do this several times alternating.

AN UNUSUAL CASE

I will relate one experience I had two years ago. The lady, a personal friend of mine, was living in the country some distance away.

I knew she had been troubled with heart attacks for several years, and it was on this account she had been obliged to retire to the quietude of a country home. When I became acquainted with the work I could do for the heart with this reflex method of massage, I wrote immediately for her to come, which she readily did. And at once I found the tender reflex, located as I have outlined it in Fig. 14.

She pleaded for mercy, and insisted I was using

47

something sharp, as a piece of glass, instead of the end of my thumb.

Finally she cried out, "Stop a minute," and said to me, "What have you done?"

I hesitated and said laughingly, "Why nothing."

She said, "Oh, yes you have," and then she went on to explain that it had felt as if a streak of lightning had flashed from her foot to her heart, followed by the sensation as if some stimulant had been administered.

I did no more at that time, but left nature to do her part.

Now to all appearances I had opened up some new channel, doing something to the circulation. For two days following she experienced a feeling of exhaustion, "just all in," as she described it, then she began to pick up. After a few more treatments the soreness had disappeared, but never again did she feel the streak of lightning effect. She gained rapidly in strength and was able to work and do things she had been denied the privilege of doing for several years, and since that time she has been able to do her work as well as anyone.

She has never had another similar heart attack.

A PHYSICIAN'S ADVICE

While relating this incident one day to a noted heart specialist, I asked Dr. B. to tell me what, in his opinion, had caused the sensation of a streak of lightning to shoot from her foot to her heart, while I was massaging that particular reflex. His reply was this. Pointing his finger at me, he said, "You obtained results didn't you? Then that is all that counts. Just keep it up."

That is exactly what I intend to do whenever I am

48

given the chance. That is why I am trying to pass this on to you that others too may be helped in the same way, and to the same extent this friend of mine has been.

ANGINA PECTORIS

I have had a number of cases of angina pectoris respond very readily to these (massage) treatments. Let me say if the pain extends up toward the shoulder and neck, work up toward the root of the fourth and fifth toes. Keep trying till you find the tenderness, then set to and work it out. I cannot lay down any stereotyped rule for you to follow, but you must work on the foot according to the location of the pain around the heart. If the pain extends down toward the arm, work around the base of the little toe, as pointed out and directed for trouble in the shoulder.

Since it is certain no harm can be done by working on a reflex, there is no need to hesitate, but set out and do all the good that can be accomplished.

With a short plump person we will find everything more compact, with one organ lying back of another, etc. and closer together than those of the taller more slender person.

THE GALL BLADDER

The gall bladder is a pear-shaped fibro muscular receptacle for the bile. Its length is from three to four inches, and its breadth about one inch. Its capacity is from eight to twelve fluid-drams and it is lined with mucous membranes. It is lodged in a fossa on the under surface of the right lobe of the liver.

GALL STONES

This we find to be a very painful trouble caused by the bile which instead of passing through the common bile duct into the duodenum, coagulates itself into hardened masses called gall stones. You can see what an important part is played here, where anything might exist causing or increasing any form of congestion.

CASE RECORD

You will be interested to hear about one particular case. Mrs. O. had been in poor health for some time. Finally it was considered necessary for her to undergo a major operation. While she was on the operating table, the doctor discovered a large stone in the gall bladder, which they considered dangerous to remove at that time because it would have kept her under an anesthetic too long. She was told she would have to return to the hospital as soon as her recovery would permit and have this stone removed.

In the meanwhile she came to me. This stone was troubling her frequently, causing severe pain attacks so that she was unable to move her arms at times. She could never reach down to pick anything up off the floor with the right arm.

I found the reflex to this sick gall bladder very tender, and believe it or not, it took only a few treatments to work out the congestion of this reflex and the pain disappeared. Fig. 15 and Fig. 16.

Now she can use her arm as well as ever; can reach up or down without the slightest discomfort, and has had no return of the pain attacks.

Mrs. O. and I often speak of this stone the doctor discovered, and we wonder what has become of it. Evidently it must have dissolved or the treatment relaxed the gall duct sufficiently so that it passed off without her knowing it.

Another case interesting to mention. Mrs. J. had experienced a number of acute gall bladder attacks, each one seemingly more severe than the one before. She could picture nothing but an operation for relief. As in all such cases, I found the reflex to the gall bladder most tender. The day following her first treatment, in the exact location of the pain center, she had a most peculiar sensation which she described as feeling like worms crawling. By stretching her body in various ways the sensation would cease for a few minutes and then return. The next day it let up gradually, and finally disappeared. This happened a year ago and Mrs. J. has had no return of the pain attacks.

If congestion causes these stones to form in the beginning, there is no telling what nature will do if we give her a chance, by relieving this congestion, which is sure to take place when the tenderness has been thoroughly worked out.

THE LIVER

The Liver is the largest gland in the body. It is located in the right side of the body and weighs about three pounds in a full grown person. Its transverse diameter is about eleven inches, its anterior posterior about eight, and its greatest vertical, five to seven inches.

It is rightly named the "King of the Glands." It is the largest organ in the body, and has within it at all times, about one-quarter of all the blood in the body circulating through it.

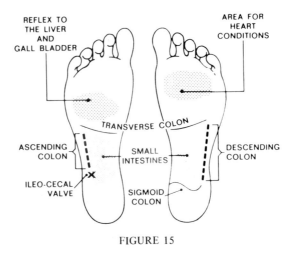

REFLEX TO
THE LIVER
AND
GALL BLADDER

AREA FOR
HEART
CONDITIONS

TRANSVERSE COLON

ASCENDING
COLON

SMALL
INTESTINES

DESCENDING
COLON

ILEO-CECAL
VALVE

SIGMOID
COLON

FIGURE 15

DIFFERENT TASKS

The Liver must perform many tasks. It manufactures bile to digest fats and prevent constipation; it is a natural antiseptic and purgative; and it helps to supply some of the substances for blood making. The liver stores up sugar within itself for future uses. It is a great filter, taking the excessive and venomous matter and waste tissues of the body and secreting and forming its own weight normally, or about two pints of bile per day. This goes into the intestines to lubricate the prevent constipation.

How necessary it is that this very important organ should function correctly, which is only possible when it receives the proper circulation.

SLUGGISH LIVER

When the liver is sluggish and fails to do its work efficiently, we must stimulate the circulation to the

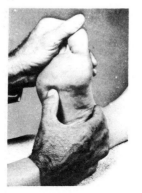

FIGURE 16
Position for Massaging the Reflex to the
Liver.

muscular tissues controlling the liver and the nerves which cause it to operate.

When we find in the foot a tenderness in the region of the reflex to the liver as shown in Fig. 15 and

Fig. 16, we know the liver is sluggish and failing to function properly.

We also know it lacks the proper circulation and muscular action necessary to keep sending the blood to the particular extremities of the feet with sufficient force to prevent a formation of crystals responsible for this tenderness in these nerve endings, which gradually increases, continuing to impede the normal circulation.

We all admit that as this condition continues over a period of days, weeks, months, and even years, we weaken the normal functions of this great important gland, and the result may be jaundice, diabetes, gall stones, atrophy, sclerosis, constipation, etc. Now as we continue massaging with a firm creeping pressure, deep into the sensitive reflex where these crystals are formed, we are able to dissolve them, lessening the obstruction so that the natural circulation can be restored. From the striking reactions we have obtained, there is no doubt of the powerful results obtainable from this ZONE THERAPY treatment.

Case Record

I will here mention the reaction in the case of Mrs. H., who had been confined to an invalid chair for six years, as the result of a severe back injury.

Being unable to exercise properly, the liver had become dormant, and even the slightest pressure caused severe pain over this region of the foot. After the third treatment this sluggish liver had received sufficient blood supply to increase its activity, and Mrs. H. had sixteen bowel movements in twenty-four hours.

EFFECTS DISCERNIBLE

You will find in every case, where a sluggish liver is involved, or any ailment resulting from this condition, that the reaction will be a tired, lifeless feeling; for nature is now struggling to combat the excessive amount of poison being eliminated from the liver during this house cleaning period. The stools at this time may be black, green, yellow or heavy mucus.

The location pointed out in these various illustrations will give you as best we can, the approximate location for a working basis. For instance, where the liver is greatly enlarged, we will find a larger portion of the foot involved. The reflex to a badly prolapsed colon will also show in a little lower position on the foot.

Case Record

Not long ago I was called to the bedside of Mr. K., age seventy-one years, who had been confined to his bed for three weeks. Several doctors had been in attendance, all expressing their opinion that Mr. K. had a very bad heart, and his weight being over three hundred pounds, none offered any hope of recovery. He had often, of late, become delirious, telling his children he had only a few more days to live.

I gave a very light treatment the first time, finding the reflex to the liver most tender. I explained the kind of reaction to expect when the circulation to that sick sluggish liver would be increased and sure enough, while the first treatment relaxed his nerves and made it possible for him to sleep without the aid of sleeping powders, the second treatment given three days later had the opposite effect.

For about twenty-four hours Mr. K. was restless, delirious, and manifesting in various ways that the increased circulation, produced by the deep massage over the reflex on the foot leading to the liver, had released the congestion, making it necessary for nature to put forth an extra effort to eliminate the excess poison.

After the third treatment given three days later, Mr. K. felt a great deal better and each treatment thereafter produced a marked improvement till he was soon up and around again.

DO NOT TREAT TOO OFTEN

If the reaction is severe, do not give another treatment too soon. Let a few days elapse to give nature a chance to adjust itself to the increased circulation.

VARICOSE VEINS

It is claimed by some that where there is a condition of varicose veins, we find trouble with the liver. Believe this or not, let me say when you have learned this method you will never be afraid of any case of varicose veins. For with the proper circulation, that congestion will disappear; just so with cramps or pains of any kind in the limbs.

THE BACK

How many people we find today who ask for some way or method of relief for a lame back.

A little study of the chart, Fig. 1, and you will acquaint yourself with the location of the zones in reference to the back.

The whole spinal column, being in the exact center of the body where the zones divide, will give us

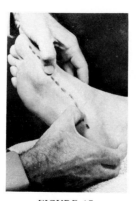

FIGURE 17

Position for Massaging the Reflex to the
Back.

the reflex for the spine in the first zone of each foot, which will cover the entire area of the inner side of the foot lengthwise from the toe to the heel.

The big toe represents that of the head; the center of the foot, the center of the back or waistline of the body; the lower part of the foot or inner part down toward the heel, the lower part of the back. See Fig. 5.

Keep this picture in your mind and it will be no trouble to find the exact location of the trouble or weakness in the back from the location of the tenderness on the inner side of the foot.

IMPINGED NERVES

The same method outlined in this book for helping other parts of the body will hold good here too. Remember every part of our body receives its nerve supply from some part of the spine, and a big majority of our ailments today can be traced to some misplacement or impinged nerve tightening the muscles of some part holding it that way with this abnormal tension.

Now since we can prove beyond a mistake or doubt that this ZONE THERAPY work on the reflexes has a definite relaxing effect, just what is going to take place as you continue to work on the reflex to the spine if it is in any way out of alignment? What will happen is this: as you relax the tension in the spinal cord your muscles will cease to contract and in the natural ways and walks of life the vertebra that was once out of alignment will often replace itself to the natural position, supplying those parts again with the proper circulation.

Congestion will take wings and fly away. The worn out depleted body cells of that part affected from this impingement will be replaced by new ones from the fresh supply of blood received now from a more perfect source of circulation.

PURE BLOOD

If you cut off any part of the blood supply to any portion of the body, you are increasing the congestion and slowing down the circulation, when circulation is the most important factor to a pure life-giving blood stream.

You are familiar with the difference between a still pool of water and a flowing stream; while the water of one becomes foul and stagnant, the other purifies itself through the oxygen in the air. Our blood purifies itself in proportion to the oxygen it picks up on its way as it passes through the lungs.

Before leaving this subject on what to do for any lameness of the back, let me relate a case record quite unusual.

CASE RECORD

Ten years ago Mrs. S. met with an automobile accident when she was thrown under the front of a truck. Lying on her back she reached forward and in some way, no one knows how, she pulled herself out from under it. In doing so she severely hurt her back. The injury was most severely deep under each shoulder blade. She soon recovered from the other minor injuries she sustained, but this pain in her back never did cease. She persistently tried every method suggested but nothing afforded relief.

Very skeptically she came to me. She was advised by a friend who came with her not to tell me where or in what part of her back the trouble existed, but to see if I could locate it from her feet. As soon as I proceeded (beginning at the top under the big toe) with this heavy pressure and began to work down, I soon reached the reflex to that part under the shoulder blades –at this point she flinched. I then knew I had found the trouble; but before asking her, I made sure there were no other tender reflexes.

Checking it carefully and finding it the same on the other foot, somewhat worse on the left than the right, I ventured to ask if her trouble might not be directly under the shoulder blades, in very deep about three to four inches from the center of the spine and worse on the left than the right side. She verified this as being exactly correct.

After a very few treatments, the trouble disappeared. There was a vivid reaction. The first night it ached severely, but the second and third treatments given every third day gradually began to bring relief till it finally disappeared entirely. She could then do her housework and use a broom to sweep for the first time since the accident.

DISORDERS OF THE KIDNEYS

The kidneys are involved in all forms of Bright's Disease, and usually in diabetic troubles.

The kidneys may be enlarged or they may be atrophied, or decreased below the normal size. They may be loosened or floated somewhat from their normal position. They may secrete either too much or not enough urine. As we have said before, any condition that is abnormal will interfere with the health of the individual. If the muscular action becomes insufficient to keep the nerve endings free from all crystalline deposits, these important organs of elimination will fail to function properly.

Now since circulation is responsible for all bodily and mental functions, and the kidneys being the eliminators of poisons from the system, the logical conclusion is that, if we can do anything to increase the circulation, we will enable the kidneys to a greater efficiency in carrying off the toxins or poisons of the system.

In dropsy it is most important to secure good and full kidney action which will at once reduce the swollen and puffed condition of the body. Where a condition of this kind exists you will be amazed at the results which can be obtained by this method of massage on the reflexes to the kidneys.

Remember we have two kidneys, one on the right side of the body and one on the left. Thus, we find the reflex to the right kidney in the right foot; the left kidney in the left foot, as shown in Fig. 5 and Fig. 19.

Since a number of ailments may result from a pair of lazy kidneys, let me say you will be surprised at how often you will find these reflexes tender. You will have astonishing results many times, even from the first treatment.

Let me warn you again, if you have a severe case of kidney trouble, do not overdo the work or treat too often, for this form of massage will have a powerful effect on the kidneys. It will take nature just so long, even with the renewed amount of circulation, to replace the old diseased kidney cells with new ones capable of sufficiently eliminating the uric acid from the system.

So just have a little patience--15 minutes every third or fourth day is often enough in most cases. For an extreme case I would suggest only once a week at first, until nature can readjust itself.

LUMBAGO

One of the most painful conditions that so often follows where the kidneys fail to do their part in eliminating the uric acid from the system is what we know as lumbago or a catch in the back.

The latest method for relief in cases of this kind is to have the patient go to bed and lie on a board for a week or two. We can imagine how this would feel when the pain is simply excruciating at even the slightest move.

But, if one is not familiar with this work on the feet, they can only hope for relief in any way suggested by the physician.

A Case Record

To relate one of my experiences in this line will explain more fully what can really be accomplished with this method of compression massage.

62

Mrs. H., apparently feeling as well as usual, was mopping her kitchen floor. As she finished, she reached over to pick up the pail and was instantly seized with this extremely painful catch in her back. She was unable to move and fell to the floor. Being alone in the house, it was nearly an hour before anyone arrived to help her up. It was impossible to get her undressed and into bed until the physician arrived to administer a sedative hypodermic injection.

Since I was out of town at the time, it was not until the following day that I could see her. She had spent a terrible night trying to lie on the ironing board. When I arrived I had to reach over the foot of the bed to work on her feet as it was impossible at first to move her feet over to the edge of the bed, as we usually do when treating a patient in bed.

I first took the right foot in my left hand and with my right thumb I began to massage the reflex to the lower part of the back as shown in Fig. 17 and 3. It was extremely tender and Mrs. H. insisted she could feel the effect of it right then in the lower end of her spine where we knew the trouble existed. I worked first on one foot then the other till the tenderness finally disappeared. By this time she could move around without the pain. For the first time since seized with this attack, she was able to move with but little pain and when I was ready to leave she got up and putting on her robe and slippers, walked into the living room. While she was still somewhat weak and shaky from the pain she had endured, the catch no longer existed and she was soon doing her work again as usual.

It is not any wonder that Mrs. H. has such a great deal of faith in what can be accomplished through massaging the reflexes of the feet; for two years ago she was suffering with diabetes, living on the strictest diet, and weighing 96 lbs. when she first came to me. Her twin sister had just passed away with this same dread disease.

I shall not try to tell you how soon she began to improve for not everyone will be able to respond so readily but, now for two years, Mrs. H. has been able to eat everything without the slightest trace of sugar showing in her urine; and today weighs 146 lbs.

If anyone is inclined to doubt this story in any way, she will be glad to have me g i v e them her name and address so she can verify what I have said.

This is only one of a number of cases I have had where a catch can be immediately relieved by thoroughly massaging the reflex to the lower lumbar region of the spine.

A little experience will help you to find the approximate location. As I have said before, if you find a tender spot, it means congestion and something which must be worked out before your patient will be one hundred percent well.

As you become accustomed to this work, if your thumbs are at all sensitive, many times it will be possible for you to feel a gritty substance as you apply the firm slow creeping massage movement with the ball of your thumb. Not in every case will you be able to feel these crystalline deposits, but I find more often with those where the muscles are firm it requires considerable pressure to find the reflexes. At least you will feel a difference at the point where the reflex is most tender. Sometimes it is in the form of a thick more solid substance which will gradually disappear as your massage work continues.

PARALYSIS

From this point let us consider the fate of one suffering from the effects of a stroke of apoplexy, the cause of which we all know to be that of a hemorrhage somewhere in the brain, usually on just one side, causing a partial or wholly paralyzed condition on the opposite side of the body to that of the head where the hemorrhage occurred.

CLOT CAUSING PRESSURE

Now consider the condition the patient is in. This tiny clot caused from the hemorrhage is causing an undue pressure on that part of the brain which governs the motor action of that half of the body which is paralyzed. The brain is unable to send a command through the delicate nerve set-up of our body and thus it remains lifeless.

Whether or not the condition will improve depends on how severe the hemorrhage has been, which we know too well all happens very suddenly and without any warning. Nevertheless, there may be a marked improvement if nature has endowed the individual with the necessary vitality to partially absorb this clot.

As the absorption of this clot takes place, it will permit a better message transference to go through from the brain to that part, the affected side, without being so heavily clouded with static. This seems to somewhat illustrate the condition that takes place.

WILL ZONE THERAPY HELP?

Now before we say whether this ZONE THERAPY method may be of any benefit to such a case, let us check back and see why this hemorrhage took place. There was a real cause, and that cause we know is generally found to be high blood pressure. Let us see if the kidneys, liver, intestines, etc. are doing their part proficiently. Unless some injury might have taken place, we know there was a cause, a primary condition responsible for this high blood pressure. This condition will still be evident after the shock, so with the information we have been giving you as to the location of the reflexes, and the stories they tell of congestion and trouble, no doubt you will soon place your finger on the keynote to the whole difficulty.

CAUSE AND EFFECT

Whatever is wrong, as the location of the tenderness will determine, set out to correct it before expecting any great improvement. Try to find and remove the cause of the high blood pressure. Then see what you can do to help the circulation of the blood to dissolve this clot as much as possible.

By doing this, you will help remove the static, thereby getting a better, a more distinct message through to the various parts of the afflicted side. We never move a finger or a toe without a message being sent through to that part from the brain guiding and directing that move, however slight it may be.

REFLEX IN THE TOES

From what has already been said regarding the various locations of the zones and reflexes, you will readily assume that the reflex to any part of the brain will be found in the big toes. Remember some of the reflexes cross at the back of the neck, so where we find the left side of the body paralyzed we may look for the reflex to this in the big toe on the right foot. Then massage the big toe on the opposite side of the body to that which is afflicted. See if any part of this toe is tender, if so work it out. By doing this you are increasing the circulation to the location of the clot in the brain, helping nature in its work of absorption. It is also advisable to massage both big toes, which will be a benefit to the whole head.

BENEFIT BY MASSAGE

One case I worked on, the whole big toe became black and blue following the treatment, and he reported feeling better by far the following day than he had at any time since his second shock a year ago. He did then recall the same toe being black and blue especially around the nail at the time of his stroke. Why it was then, and why it should be again now that I was working on it, stands out with a big question mark for you to find the answer. It was not the pressure I used that caused it either, that I know.

Let me say that the more you study along this line and begin to work on these principles for yourself, you will become more convinced every day that what I am telling you is true, and that there is still a vast field for discovery along this line of ZONE THERAPY.

SCIATICA

The great sciatica nerve supplies nearly the whole of the integument of the leg, the muscles of the back of the thigh, and of the leg and foot. It is the largest nerve cord in the body, measuring three quarters of an inch in breadth, and is the continuation of the lower part of the sacral plexus. It passes out of the pelvis through the great sacrasciatic foramen. It descends along the back part of the thigh to about its lower third, where it divides into two large branches, the internal and external popliteal nerves. It you will review your study of anatomy and examine carefully a diagram showing the posterior view of the nerves of the lower extremity, you will readily understand why this nerve can be reached through our work on the feet and on the inner side of the ankle, above and back of the ankle bone where the nerve lies nearest the surface.

Should the pressure of your thumb, as you continue to massage at this point, be too severe, try using the tip of the third finger, holding the ankle firmly in the palm of the same hand and the heel steadied with a firm grasp of the other hand. In a severe case of sciatica, where the inflammation has been of long standing, do not be surprised if the first few treatments bring tears to the eyes of your patient. To prevent this if possible, watch carefully the expression, so as to quickly let up as soon as you feel you have gone the limit of what the patient can stand. Here you must use care and let the pressure of the massage be gradual, and steadily increase as the pain subsides.

WHAT CAUSES SCIATICA

Sciatica is generally accepted as the result of some misplacement along the lumbar region. But we find, too, there can be other causes for this painful malady, such as an enlargement of the prostate gland or injury to some other part of the body affecting the sciatic nerve.

Case Record

It was a case of this type I had the pleasure of relieving a short time ago. Mr. P., a man about 55 years of age, came to me with but little faith in his heart that I would be able to help his case with my method of work on his feet. For eight years he had suffered untold agony. He had been confined to his bed for days and weeks at a time, and he had spent a small fortune as you can imagine any one would do in such a painful condition, visiting the very best and most reputable physicians the medical or drugless profession had to offer. The question remained, would I be able to locate, in my simple way, the cause and relief for this exceptionally stubborn case. I decided it could be no misplacement in the lumbar region as that would have been corrected long ago. I reasoned that the cause in this case was different. I would be sure to find a formation of crystals in that great nerve ending somewhere in the foot and leg that had failed to respond to any other form of treatment. As I proceeded with the end of my thumb, the slow creeping rotary massage of that part of the foot as shown in Fig. **17,** reflex for the lower lumbar region, there was no longer a question as to the congestion in the lumbar area. I proceeded up the inside and outside of the ankle, above and back of the ankle bone, till I found more and more of these crystals. Even the slightest pressure and massage in these regions caused intense pain.

After about twenty minutes work on the affected side and ten minutes working alternately on the other foot, which was also somewhat tender, Mr. P. arose and in walking around could immediately feel some relief. After several treatments given every third day, there was a decided improvement, especially the day following each treatment. As I became impatient for somewhat quicker results, Mr. P. would constantly remind me that his was a case of eight years standing, and that I was already doing more for him than anyone else had done.

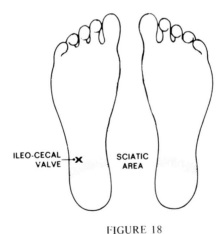

FIGURE 18

One evening, having a little spare time after the treatment, I set out to question Mr. P. to see if I might determine the cause. Calling to mind the rules of ZONE THERAPY, and the reflex relation of one part of the body to the other as taught by Dr. Fitz-Gerald, I inquired if he might at any time in the past have injured his shoulder, or arm on that afflicted side. This he heartily confirmed by showing me how impossible it was to raise that arm properly, it having been broken and improperly set, then rebroken several times, endeavoring to remedy the first injury. This had happened four or five years before the sciatic trouble had set in. Now the question arises: Could these injured nerves in the shoulder have any reflex action in the hip that could lessen the normal circulation of the great sciatic nerve, or will we say cause a short circuit in some way? We leave you to guess. We do know something had certainly impeded the circulation, burning off the insulation to cause so much inflammation and discomfort.

The extreme tenderness in that foot meant an exag-gerated formation of crystals that had gradually been increasing as the trouble continued.

Let the cause be what it may, I found certain parts of the shoulder very tender, which I thoroughly massaged. Then to help this I returned to the reflex in the foot leading to the shoulder as shown in Fig. 20 and Fig. 21 and Fig. 22, which was also very tender. With all these forces brought to bear, it was only a reasonable time till Mr. P. was entirely free from every particle of pain. It is my candid belief that his whole trouble had its origin in that injury to his shoulder.

When inflammation of this great sciatic nerve exists, we can readily understand why it would be a most painful and soul-racking disease. But it can be easily relieved by the simple method we herein set forth, if accompanied with persistent effort and a little patience, which is the only way to accomplish anything worth while.

BURSITIS

While we are calling your attention to the location on the foot having a reflex action on the shoulder, let me tell you what can be done for many a lame aching shoulder, that may have refused to respond to other forms of treatment.

I recall a case of bursitis. The young lady, a telephone operator, had been disabled for nearly a year.

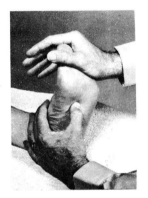

FIGURE 19

Position for Massaging the Reflex to
the Kidneys

It was impossible to raise the arm more than a few inches from her body. She was discouraged for nothing yet had offered any relief. Many forms of heat and electricity had been applied, which only increased the pain.

Now we know in any case of bursitis we are handling inflammation of the bursa, and until this inflammation has subsided, it is not advisable to massage directly over the afflicted part. Then let us concentrate our efforts on the reflex to this shoulder as pointed out in Fig. 20.

You will find--as we shall call it--the root of the little toe representing that of the shoulder, and as you press firmly in and around that area you will find some extremely tender spot which can be worked out in time, having a definite effect on the afflicted shoulder without any direct contact with the shoulder itself.

CAUSES OF BURSITIS

In a case of this kind we must always look for what might be the cause of bursitis, neuritis, rheumatism, or such kindred ailments. See if the kidneys are not lazy and refusing to throw off the uric acid sufficiently to prevent an acid condition of the blood, as was definitely the cause of the case I just mentioned. This young lady was being treated for Bright's Disease at the time she came to my office. As I proceeded to massage the reflex to the kidneys, which was extremely sensitive, the kidney action increased, and this in turn cleared the system of that excessive acid condition. In a few weeks the back ceased to ache and pain, as it had done for some time. The arm loosened up and she was able to raise it a few inches higher after each treatment. She was soon able to resume her duties at the switchboard and has been feeling fine ever since.

NEURITIS OF THE SHOULDER

I could fill many pages relating the various experiences encountered where the arm and shoulder were lame from some form of neuritis. It may be interesting to relate my experience with one of these.

Case Record

Mr. S. while at his work, fell on a slippery floor, causing a severe injury to his shoulder. He had several X-rays taken which proved there were no broken bones, but the pain grew worse till at the end of three weeks he was unable to sleep without a sedative for the severe pain. He could not raise or move his arm, and he came to me with tears in his eyes as he was suffering so severely and dreaded to see night coming on when it always seemed worse. It was his right shoulder, so I took the right foot and without any further ceremony, reached for the part leading to his lame shoulder. I will admit the tears did not let up, but simply increased as he pleaded for mercy, not that I was harsh or rough, but the tenderness was so extreme even to the slightest touch. As I worked on it, the pain, however, soon let up.

In a case of this kind it is best to work two or three minutes, then rest a little and meanwhile try to convince the patient that this tenderness in his foot is there as a reflex from that experienced in his shoulder, as you want him to be patient with you and your work for fifteen or twenty minutes. Let your conversation be cheerful and constructive to keep his mind off what you are doing as much as possible. In the meantime you are holding his right foot in your left hand using your right thumb for the pressure and massage; as you steady the pressure with your fingers on the top of the foot as in Fig. 20.

Keep working around this joint of the little toe and watch the improvement. By this time he will most likely be able to raise his arm up over his head, as did Mr. S. and it was less than a week when he was able to go back to work.

It is most interesting to work on such cases. Your efforts will be rewarded so quickly and results will be lasting.

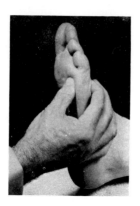

FIGURE 20
Position for Massaging the Reflex to the Shoulder.

A BROKEN SHOULDER

Case Record

Let me mention here also a case where the shoulder had been broken in an automobile accident, both the clavical and scapula were broken within an inch of the glenoid cavity, and the humerous was cracked.

The patient, a physician about seventy years of age, was taken to the hospital as he also received a broken leg just below the knee and three fractured ribs, all on the left side. The leg was placed in a cast and the shoulder in a specially formed brace.

He called for me soon after all parts, casts, etc., had been set and adjusted. The part for the shoulder on his left foot, was just at the edge of the cast leaving it possible for me to do my part on the reflex for the broken shoulder, which by now was already most tender.

Since he was in such a weakened condition from the seriousness of the accident, it was advisable that I do only a little at a time and that more often. At first I worked it gently a little every day then every second day. It was remarkable to watch the speed of his recovery and the excellent use he soon regained of the arm and shoulder.

It is evident, this method of reflex massage used on that particular reflex hastened the progress and healing of those broken bones by increasing the circulation and relieving the congestion.

TO LOOSEN THE MUSCLES OF THE SHOULDER

We find a large majority of people suffering more or less from a tired feeling across the back of the neck and shoulders. To help relieve this nervous tension, press firmly with the knuckles against the sole of the foot while you massage and loosen up the cords and muscles across the top of the foot as shown in Fig. 21.

These will be extremely tight where the patient is nervous and high strung. In such a case do not neglect to massage this part thoroughly on each foot, for it will prove a very important factor in bringing about relief from many ailments caused by undue nerve tension.

To massage this part of the foot is also very essential where there is any tendency to a broken metatarsal arch. If this condition has existed very long, you must be persistent with this part of the massage work in order to break up and loosen any calcium deposits which may have formed around the joints which have become misplaced.

If any one or more of the 26 bones of the foot should be misplaced, nature fills in that misplaced joint with a calcium deposit which we can help to loosen and dissolve by this form of massage over the top of the foot as shown in Figure 21, and also the twisting movement as illustrated in Figure 26.

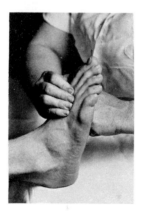

FIGURE 21

Position for Loosening the Muscles of the
Shoulder and Neck

You will readily see how this will help nature to carry away any such foreign matter which interferes with the normal position of the bones.

A LAME HIP

Keep in mind this reflex in the shoulder where there is a condition in any part of the hip.

Since a reflex can be found in the shoulder for the hip, let us remember that to loosen up any part of the shoulder will have a tendency to relieve tightness and congestion in the hip. It will require a very deep pressure as illustrated in Fig. 21 and Fig. 20

Should the pain extend below the hip between that and the knee, massage deeply that part of the arm between the shoulder and the elbow; any heavy deep massage given around the shoulder and back of the neck will help relieve any tightness or congestion in the corresponding part of the hip.

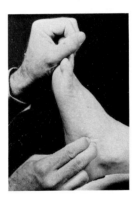

FIGURE 22

Position for Loosening the Muscles relative
to Hip and Shoulder.

It is also well to remember the same rule holds good with the shoulder. Many times a pain there can be relieved by a heavy deep massage of the corresponding part in the hip itself. Be sure to work the reflex to the hips as shown in Fig. 22.

ARTHRITIS

Arthritis is a condition from which many are seeking relief. Like every other ailment there must be a cause. If that cause is an infection brought about by food poisoning, let us see why the digestive system is lazy and fails to function normally.

The time occupied for a normal meal to pass through the digestive system (stomach and intestines) is from twelve to eighteen hours, but if these organs are weakened by a congestion in the nerve endings (in the feet), then the stomach fails to function properly.

Food supposed to be acted upon in the stomach, if not properly prepared for its reception into the intestines, ferments and decomposes. The blood, which is dependent upon the material handed to it from the digestive organs, is overloaded with acid or calcium deposits. As this condition increases the vitality of the body decreases leaving the patient subject to arthritis, rheumatism, neuritis, etc. Thus if you will seek to find the cause from "The Stories the Feet Can Tell," you will most likely find which organ or organs might be mainly responsible for this condition and, as in everything else, if we can remove the cause we help the effect. Do not look for results in arthritis in a minute, a day or a week. It will take time. They will most likely feel somewhat worse from the first few treatments due to the reaction, but do not become impatient for results. As long as the slightest tenderness remains in the nerve endings in the feet, you are still fighting to break up and scatter crystalline deposits.

CIRCULATION AND CONSTIPATION

Increased circulation can become a powerful house-cleaning agent, and thus stimulate a rectal action in a normal regular rhythm without the use of drugs or the regular old fashioned enema with which in olden times people prided themselves in the number of gallons of water they could use, and the length of time

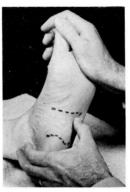

FIGURE 23
Position for Massaging the Reflex to the Colon.

it took to perform this bowel cleansing. At times it has been known that three to eight gallons of water were used and an hour and a half of time consumed.

We all admit that in cases of acute autointoxication, this method of immediate relief might be necessary, and be used to great advantage. But where the present condition has already existed over a period of time without any serious effects except ordinary discomfort, we can afford to give nature a little time to adjust its elimination, and thus allow the large bowel to serve the useful purpose nature intended it should, by absorbing through its walls some of the water and certain necessary minerals which are returned to the body after entering it from the small intestines. At this point it is in somewhat of a liquid state. As the absorption takes place, the contents of the large lower bowel becomes semi-solid, and to help this mass to pass on with the normal muscular action of the bowels, it must become lubricated with mucus secreted by the intestinal glands, and finally it reaches the rectum almost solid.

Here we need proper contraction of the muscles in the walls of the large bowel to call the attention of the person to the fact that he is ready for a movement.

You can readily see that any change in this program brought about by the habitual use of a purgative or an irritating enema, will change the natural routine nature mapped out. Don't try to improve on God's natural laws of nature. It is only as we abuse these precious laws that we suffer from the many ills mankind has fallen heir to.

RELAXING EFFECT

SOME CASES OF CONSTIPATION

It is very evident from the results we obtain, that this treatment, this method of massage has a definite relaxing influence on the part being treated through the reflex. You will come to the same conclusion with me, after having a few experiences similar to what I have had in some cases of constipation.

CONSTIPATION AND CONTRACTION

Now since the cause of this prevailing ailment is often due to a contraction or tension of some form of the lower bowel, we find that to thoroughly massage the part on the inner side of each ankle, beginning from the heel and working up about six or eight inches, will often produce an immediate bowel movement. For location see Fig. 24 .

The position of the hands in giving this treatment is the same as described for disorders of the rectum.

We can also emphasize this effect by loosening up the tendon of Achilles, the cord leading up the back of the leg from the heel. You may do this while the foot is still in the firm grasp of your hand. It will feel much like a firm rubber cord. While you are using the tips of your fingers for the other work we have described, do not fail at the same time to press this cord back and forth in any way that might tend to stretch it and relieve any form of tightness, hold the ankle firmly while twisting the foot as shown in Fig. 26.

JUST WHEN TO EXPECT IMMEDIATE RESULTS

Do not misunderstand me and say I claim that every form of constipation can be relieved by this method. I qualified it, in the beginning of this chapter, when I said some cases of constipation are due to nerve tension affecting and tightening the sphincter muscles of the rectum causing undue contraction of the sigmoid flexure.

It is with cases of this origin we so often obtain immediate results. It is nothing unusual to have someone come into my office, and rave about how much good I have done for them and their particular case of constipation. Perhaps since the first treatment (massage) they have been able to discard the use of their daily cathartic, while the neighbor next door may fail to respond till the whole intestinal tract, liver, and gall bladder have been brought into proper action.

LENGTH OF TIME

The length of time for results in a case of this kind will depend entirely on just how long they have been in getting out of tune, or whether they may have had one or more operations to impede the progress of this repair work. Perhaps, too, they have had their appendix removed, robbing the intestines of that little oil supply so important to the normal action of the bowels.

We who have been fortunate enough to escape any such operation, robbing us of any organ of our body, however small or insignificant it may seem, have just that much more for which to be thankful. We will also be in a condition to respond more readily to ZONE THERAPY treatments.

RECTAL DISORDERS

It is astonishing the results that can be obtained from this treatment for various disorders of the rectum. We will first give you the location of this reflex. Stop and think and in your mind's eye decide in which zone the rectum is located. Being in the center of the body, places it in the first zone. Therefore, we will find this reflex on the inner side of each ankle about half an inch from the cord leading up the back of the leg, shown in Fig. 24.

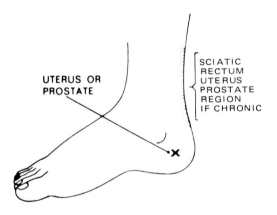

UTERUS OR
PROSTATE

SCIATIC
RECTUM
UTERUS
PROSTATE
REGION
IF CHRONIC

SAME REFLEX AREAS
FOUND ON BOTH FEET

FIGURE 24

The tenderness here may extend three to five inches up from the heel, according to the amount and location of the trouble in the rectum, which varies in length from six to eight inches.

This will be found extremely tender, wherever there is an inflamed or abnormal condition of the rectum.

PROSTATE GLAND

We find the location of this important gland, which resembles that of a horsechestnut in form and size, is in the first zone, since it surrounds the neck of the bladder and commencement of the urethra, lying in the pelvic cavity behind and below the symphisis pubis upon the rectum. An enlargement of this gland will cause considerable pain and inconvenience and often

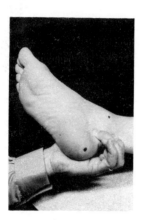

FIGURE 25

Position for Massaging the Reflex to the
Prostate Gland on both feet.

results in a great deal of difficulty in voiding the urine. It affects the nervous system and is oftentimes responsible for the patient being aroused a number of times during the night to urinate.

Wherever this condition exists you will be sure to find this reflex to the rectum very tender, perhaps extending down to the lower part of the inside of the heel toward that of the bladder. Lying so closely together it is impossible to separate the reflex, but you will find a tenderness here at this point to tell of the congestion to that particular part or gland which is causing the inflammation or irritation.

AN ENLARGED PROSTATE GLAND

First find the location as per Figs. 24 and 25.

After locating the tenderness, grasp the foot according to directions given for treating disorders of the rectum. Continue the pressure and creeping massage with the thumb or finger tips, using whichever seems the best way to work out and dissolve the crystal-like substance that has accumulated in that particular nerve ending, caused by the inflammation and enlargement of the gland.

Remember you are endeavoring to restore the normal circulation without any direct contact which would tend to set up an increased irritation. There has been a cause for this gland to grow into a diseased state, and that cause was no doubt a congestion brought about by the crystals in these nerve endings.

Now let us consider how we can cause this gland to grow out of this diseased condition. Certainly there is no better or more effective way to do this, than to supply the parts again with the amount of free and normal circulation nature intended they should have.

Case Record

To prove this statement I shall relate a case that came to my attention a little while ago. Mr. V., a man about 50 years of age, had been having treatments for an enlarged prostate gland, with little or no results. I proceeded at once with this compression massage in the manner as shown in Fig. 25. I found as I always do in such cases, a great deal of tenderness in the reflex to the prostate gland. But after the tenderness had been completely worked out we found the trouble had entirely disappeared, and instead of being disturbed from four to six times each night to urinate, he was able to rest undisturbed for eight or ten hours.

Now at this time there happened a most interesting coincidence. For some time Mr. V. had been conscious that a small growth had formed just inside at the end of the rectum which he was very anxious to have removed. Since he was now feeling in the pink of condition he thought it a most opportune time to have this slight operation performed.

The treatments (massaging) I had given him had completely cleared up all the tenderness of that part, and relieved all undue congestion from the prostate gland. His nervousness had improved too. The night before the operation we tested it out thoroughly to assure ourselves that not the slightest tenderness anywhere remained.

Then I arranged to see Mr. V. again as soon as possible following the operation. At this time I knew we would find an exaggerated amount of tenderness in the lower part of the ankle as the result of the operation, which as I explained to to Mr. V. would be a splendid test as to the accuracy of my statements, and the location of the reflexes.

When I arrived he had only been home a few hours from the doctor's office. He was in considerable pain with the rectum aching and throbbing and feeling very uncomfortable. I immediately found the reflex with the tip of my third finger, and to him it felt, under the slightest pressure, as if I were piercing it with a piece of broken glass; the same place and tenderness showing up on each ankle.

It is evident the removal of this growth directly on the rectum, which is in the center of the body, had affected the first zone on each side.

I proceeded with a gentle massage on first one ankle, then the other, alternating about every two minutes for about a quarter of an hour. The throbbing soon disappeared and it was amazing the amount of relief this gave him and so soon, even following an operation. He was able at once to turn over in bed without pain, and was up and around as usual in a short time.

HEMORRHOIDS

We will now consider a case of hemorrhoids (commonly called piles). This is a condition of varicose veins (congestion) in the rectum, causing very great tenderness and inconvenience, and sometimes bleeding. It is on account of this tenderness in the region of the rectum that we find the reflex to the rectum so sensitive, indicating a congestion preventing the circulation.

ONE POSITION FOR TREATING HEMORRHOIDS

As you sit facing the patient, first place the left heel in your left hand, grasp the leg with your right hand just above the ankle from the under side. With the tips of your fingers pointing upward, hold the foot steady with your left hand. You must use the right hand to massage firmly with a rotary motion, till you locate the tenderest spot, and there continue with your pressure, and massaging in the same way and in the same place as that outlined for disorders of the rectum on Pg. 84. Reverse the procedure on the right heel.

NOT TOO MUCH PRESSURE

You must use caution not to be too severe, the nerves being close to the surface at this point. It will require time and patience more than severity.

Let me say again, you must watch the expression of your patient carefully to determine just where and when you are reaching the point that will produce the desired effect (tenderness). So often the beginner will keep watching his hands. Learn to let the hands automatically hunt and find the sore places without trying to look at them. It is far more important to watch the expression attentively, which helps you to determine how much pressure can be used without causing too much pain.

You are not trying to do the work all in a minute, It will require time. As you see the distress signal on the face of the patient, caused by what you are doing, you can let up quickly and proceed more gently and can also locate your reflex more correctly. This reflex may cover only an area as large as a pea, and sometimes even less.

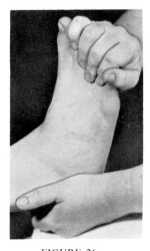

FIGURE 26

Method of Twisting Foot for Relief of
Congestion in General.

In a condition of hemorrhoids you will find a tightness of the heavy cord leading up the back of the leg, which may be loosened up considerably by twisting the foot around in a circulatory motion three or four times to the right, then alternating three or four times to the left, pulling the heel and stretching the cord by pressing the foot forward and pulling it backward. This can be done best while the foot is still in this position. with the heel resting on your hand.

I want to say here that before giving this twist you must change the grasp of your right hand to that of the top of the foot, as shown in Fig. 26. The more pressure placed by the heel of your right hand against the sole of the foot, at the location of the metatarsal arch, while twisting the foot, the greater the tendency to loosen up the bones and correct any slight misplacement that might exist in that particular arch. This work done faithfully twice a week allowing about one half hour for each treatment till all tenderness had disappeared will practically remove all discomfort and annoyance caused by any case of hemorrhoids.

CASE RECORD

It may be interesting here to relate an experience I had in Miami, Florida, a few years ago. I was explaining this method of treating, and how we could locate the reflex to the rectum etc. to a small group of friends, when a young lady stepped forward whom I had never met before and offered herself as a subject for me to use in demonstrating this ZONE THERAPY.

Her outward appearance was that of perfect health, so I began the examination in the usual way, wondering if I would be able to find any tender reflex to indicate any weakness in one so apparently healthy.

Beginning at the big toe I proceeded with the usual pressure on each of the principal reflexes of the foot, without the slightest response to indicate any tenderness or bodily ailment. But as I grasped the ankle and began to press on the point which would indicate some rectal disorder, or most likely hemorr-

hoids, she almost jumped out of the chair and exclaimed, "Oh, that hurts!"

Knowing I had located some ailment or weakness
I went on to ask the young lady if she might have
had any trouble in that line recently. Before answering me, she smiled as if to ask, how did I know -
then went on to tell that only a few weeks before, she
had undergone the third operation for hemorrhoids
and had not yet entirely recovered.

She was most thoroughly convinced with the truthfulness of my remarks. What interested us all still
further was the story she went on to tell. As she was
"coming to" from the effects of the ether given for her
last operation, before gaining consciousness, she had
to be strapped to the bed to prevent her from constantly
rising up and grabbing her heels and crying, "Oh,
how my heels hurt."

KNOWLEDGE OF "ZONE THERAPY"

With the knowledge we have now of the zones and
reflexes of the body we can readily understand why
nature was calling out in despair at the damage done
to some part of that elementary nerve canal zone.
While the mind was still in that state of semi-conscious-
ness, the sub-conscious mind was working and calling
for pressure to that reflex as a form of relief.

Had the nurses in that hospital understood ZONE
THERAPY and instead of strapping her down in bed,
had administered a little pressure and light massage
to that region of her heel, it would have given this poor
girl a great deal of relief, and would have aided the
process of recovery by increasing the circulation to
the wounded area.

Suffice to say, from this demonstration the young lady was a firm believer in ZONE THERAPY. She placed herself in my care for a while and she was soon feeling fit and fine as ever.

PROLAPSED RECTUM

Case Record

As further evidence of what can really be accomplished by work of this kind I will relate a case I had the pleasure of caring for in my own family.

A lady over 70 years of age, since the birth of her daughter some 30 years ago, had been troubled terribly with a prolapsed rectum. Each year as she grew older, it became worse and protruded more and more. A greater portion of the time it would be swollen badly and very much inflamed.

A number of physicians had suggested an operation, as a means of the only possible relief, it being very likely to produce even a more serious form of trouble by destroying the muscular action of the rectum for all future time.

Knowing a little experimentation on my part with our Zone Therapy work would do no harm, I set out to see what I could do. The results and the benefit that she received from a few of these massage treatments were almost unbelievable. The inflammation and swelling subsided entirely, and it has caused her little or no trouble since. I simply used the method I have outlined for disorders of the rectum and hemorrhoids on Page 84.

Let me say here that in this case the tenderness was extremely manifest and many times she would plead for mercy during the treatment, when in reality the pressure was in no way severe. But as the tenderness gradually worked out the condition improved.

INFLAMMATION OF THE BLADDER

CYSTITIS

Inflammation of the bladder causing a frequent desire to urinate, is a condition very easy to handle with this form of massage treatment. The reflex is found on each foot, in practically the same location as outlined for the lower part of rectum only a little more

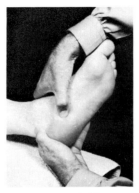

FIGURE 27

Method for Massaging the Reflex to the
Bladder

toward and under the ankle bone as in Fig. 27. The bladder and rectum being in so nearly the same (first) zone. This works out quickly, perhaps the second or third treatment will show a marked improvement, together with your work on the kidneys which will help to lessen the formation of uric acid which no doubt originally caused by cystitis.

TENSION OF FEMALE ORGANS

UTERUS

It is with this same mode of treatment that you will be able to help many a trouble caused by a tension or a tightening of the muscles of the uterus and vagina. This condition is responsible for a great deal of nervousness and the breaking up of many a happy home.

When a case of this kind is brought to your attention, think a little of what might be the cause and effect, and set out to remedy it. Perhaps you will be able to steer more than one unhappy individual from the rocks of disaster.

OVARIES

Now picture in your mind the location of the ovaries. They are located somewhat away from the center and each one off to the side a little. Thus we will find the reflex to the right ovary on the outside of the right heel, and the left ovary reflected on the outside of the left heel. Fig. 28.

Where the thyroid gland is affected in any way, you will most likely find this point tender too, as the thyroid gland is considered sort of a third ovary, and connected very closely in their relationship to the functioning of the monthly period.

I could relate some wonderful results I have had

in this line, where the irregularity was caused by an abnormal functioning of the thyroid gland.

Case Record

One case I remember in particular, a young lady 35 years old had never menstruated regularly since maturity. Instead of the normal period every twenty-eight days she was always exactly forty days between her periods. She had since childhood been subject to severe attacks of hives, considered most likely the result of a nervous disturbance of some form. Finally she began to lose interest in her home, did not care to live, lost weight rapidly, went down

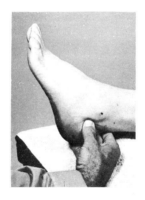

FIGURE 28

Position for Massaging the Left Ovary.

from 130 lbs. to about 90 lbs.

She was taken to the hospital for observation. Tests showed a case of exophthalmic goitre. She was ordered to return home and build up for the operation they advised. She came to me at this time.

I found a great deal of nerve tension and congestion present in the location just outlined for ailments of this kind. She was persuaded to postpone the operation and give me a chance to see what could be done with this reflex work.

Improvement was noticeable almost immediately from the beginning of the treatments. Her nerves improved, she grew more calm every day, rested better, and as I recall, it was only two or three weeks till she began to gain weight regularly, about one pound a week, till she was again back to normal, feeling like herself and in splendid condition. She was now for the first time in her life normal and regular in her monthly periods, proving what I am trying to bring out, that a sick thyroid will affect the functioning of the ovaries.

You will often be asked if with this method of compression massage you can do anything to relieve cramps during the menstruation period. In a case where the cause is congestion you will get surprising results. We all know there may be a variety of causes for a condition of this kind.

While we do not claim this method to be any form of magic, or a cure-all for every ailment let us not fail to give it credit for what we know it can do for such a large variety of cases. Let us consider a case of hemorrhage. I would say, by all means, do not give this treatment during that period, unless guided and directed by a competent physician familiar with the case and familiar with the results obtainable from this Reflex Therapy treatment.

RESULTS WILL FOLLOW

By your persistent endeavor you will be sure to obtain results, and these various ailments will finally disappear. Not over night, nor in a day, or a week, as you must remind the patient, this is not a faith cure performed by wielding some magic wand over the head, but a scientific method worked out on scientific principles.

Our body is constructed to endure a lot of abuse. We have been breaking the laws of nature over a period of months and years, and it will take time to rebuild and replace these sick broken down cells.

We are inclined to give the working of our automobile more thought and consideration than we do our precious body. We take it to a garage every now and then for a check-up, to see that every bolt and nut is tight, and that every part is properly lubricated, even the slightest rattle or squeak receives our immediate attention. But when a pain attacks us here and there, as a warning of some impending danger, we try to brush it aside and say, "Oh, it will wear off." Sometimes it will, all well and good, again it may wear us out during the procedure.

How many can we recall who have gone to an earlier grave than necessary because they neglected the danger signal in time to avert the fatal accident, which might have at least been postponed for several years, with a little added attention given to the congested areas of their body?

We must remember circulation is life; stagnation is death; a heavy blow causes congestion, and tenderness is the result. Just so with any part of the body starved by congestion in any part of the zone leading to that particular muscle or organ of the body.

REFLEXES OTHER THAN FOUND IN THE FEET

From the teachings set forth and brought out on ZONE THERAPY by Doctor FitzGerald, we have learned, too, of other reflexes than those found in the feet, which have a lot to do with one being successful in this great cause; a knowledge of which when combined with this work on the feet, can bring relief to many a swollen aching joint.

We who are trained in the science of massage, know very well how often it is inadvisable to massage directly over an aching swollen part, for if a condition of neuritis (inflammation of the nerves) should exist, we might aggravate the trouble and increase the pain. But if we are familiar with the location of the reflex to that particular part in another place on the body, we can massage this most thoroughly and have a definite effect on the afflicted area.

Suppose someone comes to you with neuritis in the right knee. You will take the right elbow, and in the exact location on the elbow as that of the trouble in the knee, you will find a tenderness. Massage this deeply with the thumb and tips of your fingers, reaching in to loosen up the ligaments, tendons, etc. After keeping this up for perhaps ten minutes, then ask if any improvement is noticed in the condition of the knee; invariably it will be noticeable immediately.

Now if the trouble is in the elbow, we massage the knee on the same side, which will have a reflex action on the elbow.

We find the wrist can be successfully massaged for troubles in the ankle; the right wrist for the right ankle, the left wrist for the left ankle. As in the knee and the elbow so the tenderness will be found in the wrist, in exact proportion corresponding to the location of the tenderness in the ankle.

A STIFF OR LAME SHOULDER

A lame shoulder which will have a particular point of tenderness, can be reached by locating this same point in the hip and working directly on that part of the hip.

A stiffness caused by adhesions following a broken hip, can be greatly improved by deep heavy massage of every muscle in the shoulder on that particular side.

The same method will hold good with a case where the shoulder has been broken, remaining stiff and lame from the effects of a cast or adhesions and such like.

It may be impossible to move the arm, yet the leg and hip on that side can be moved without causing any discomfort. So the work you would like to be doing on the arm and shoulder itself, to loosen it up, but find yourself unable to on account of the stiffness, you can do to the leg and hip on that side and watch the results. You will not be causing any pain yet producing an effect impossible to get by any direct contact with the part itself.

A few experiences in this line will increase your faith and confidence in what can be done with reflex work. Some improvements will be observed and felt almost immediately, which encourages both the patient and the operator, and increases faith all around in the effectiveness of what is being done. You may not have to wait for results when you use this method for trouble in the joints, etc.

MIND AND DIGESTION

The state of mind affects digestion more than almost any other bodily ailment.

Constipation is often a state of the mind. Dr. Boris Kaplan has published recent studies indicating that financial troubles may cause stomach disorders, which become ulcers. The worries affect the digestion, and the digestive troubles increase the worry. Thus a case refusing to respond to the usual form this foot treatment, may be traced to some emotional disturbance in the patient's life.

I will relate a case here that was brought to my attention. Mrs. H., about 45 years of age, came to me for treatments. Her husband was a very successful business man and had always been a good provider. She had a comfortable home, a cottage at the lake in the summer, and four nice children, youngest still in high school. But in spite of it all, she developed a complex which led her to believe she was sick. She visited several physicians, who with X-rays and various tests, could discover nothing wrong with her condition, for which they were heartily condemned. Her husband, frantic to find help, brought her to me, as a last resort, and as I began to explain my method of finding a tenderness in the reflex of the foot, leading to the affected part, she began to tell me she knew she had colitis, and ulcers of the stomach. She couldn't eat, she couldn't sleep, and she knew she was going to lose her mind if something could not be done for her.

From the sound of her story I expected to find a

number of tender places. As I now proceeded with the usual pressure, to my surprise I too found nothing to indicate any calcium or crystal deposits, which would instead prove a very healthy condition, verifying the physician's diagnosis. Her husband, believing my method to be his last resort, insisted I try to convince her that it would be of some help. On each visit, she would assure me she was going to lose her mind, as she was so very sick. I used all the power of suggestion that was possible to bring to bear, but to no avail. Nothing I could do helped her because there was no real trouble to correct, except the mental complex which was so deeply rooted in her mind, that she brought upon herself the very mental condition she feared. And in a short time it was necessary to confine her to the State Hospital, where she has been for the last two years.

How pitiful to see anyone bring about such a condition simply from a distorted mental attitude, when no real physical ailment existed. Without a doubt, Mrs. H. attracted to herself, that which she actually feared. As we continue our study along this line, we find that most bodily ailments affect us in proportion as we give them attention.

There is not an organ in the body that is not affected by the mind. Every thought we think either has a constructive or a destructive reaction on the chemical content of our blood stream. We cannot let thoughts of fear, worry, anxiety or grief overcome us without increasing the acidity of our bloodstream. Worry is a magnified form of fear, an idea by which we torment ourselves, a fixation of attention.

How often our health is controlled by fixed ideas. Most of our nervous derangements are brought on by uncontrolled emtions. A suggestion can sometimes prove a power to determine a destiny. Are we going to let thoughts of fear kill the cells of our body? How many times have we seen the seriousness of an epidemic increased by the fear thoughts that invaded the minds of the people? The twenty-seven trillion cells of the body all have their thinking machine, and they all respond to the law of suggestion. It is the law of creation, and we cannot tamper with it.

CIRCULATION FOLLOWS ATTENTION

A doctor who breezes into a sick room with a cheerful disposition, can do a world of good for his patient, and can start the creative powers to work, or he can have the opposite effect; for those who are down and sick are always susceptible to suggestion.

It is an acknowledged fact that the body is affected by the mind. Every flitting change of the mind causes a chemical change in the body. Circulation follows attention. We are told that the center of every cell in the body is composed of the same grey matter as the brain. Every time we think a thought, we use up energy. Then why continue to poison our system and waste our energies by harboring destructive thoughts of fear, worry, envy, jealousy and their kindred folks? We cannot change a natural law. It takes certain laws and principles to make us free from disease. And the more we learn of the truth about these laws of nature, that rule and govern our health--which too are also God's laws--the quicker our system becomes freed from these destructive agencies, and we no longer continue in such a way as to tear down our body cells.

MIND AND DEMAND

Our mind can change a demand. Our ideals can be changed by a new thought. Some authorities go so far as to claim that cancer can be caused by a long continuous nerve retention. That gall bladder trouble can be brought on by anxiety; that secretive nervous irritation can cause fibroid tumor; and constipation can be brought on by obstinacy, and some forms of rheumatism to be a state of unconscious unwillingness to face the problems of life. Whether this will all be true or not, we mention it for your consideration. No doubt the predominant mental impression is what governs the mind and the functioning of every part of our being even to the tiniest cell.

CRYSTALLINE DEPOSITS

This in turn has to do with governing the acid content in our bloodstream, and the amount of crystals that may be liable to form in the nerve ending of any organ of the body that might be unable to do its part in keeping up with the normal muscular action necessary to keep the circulation normally perfect.

If the gas line in our automobile becomes choked up in any way, the carburetor ceases to function properly, and the power dies down. Then we must go to a garage, and employ the aid of someone trained in locating the obstruction to eliminate it.

ACID DEPOSITS

This corresponds exactly with the work we are aiming to do to these acid deposits in the nerve endings of the feet. We must clear the gas line (arteries and veins) of any foreign obstruction, before the carburetor (heart) can work proficiently and furnish the body sufficient power and pep to perform its round of duty as nature intended it should. Since we cannot exchange this old body for a new model every year, it is all the more necessary that we give special attention to the one and only one we can ever own.

OUR BODY A MACHINE

This machine, our body, is one thing left to our care, and if we abuse it, the sooner it will wear out.

If we allow calcium deposits to increase in our arteries after the age of forty, we are soon having high blood pressure, overburdening the heart in its effort to keep the blood in circulation even to the tiniest nerve extremities of the hands and feet.

WHAT IS PAIN?

Pain is not a disease, but it is a true indication of a disturbance, a congestion in some part or parts. Pain is not an evil but a blessing, calling out for help; a cry of nature. Then why try to deaden the warning call by the use of aspirin or some sedative which will only tend to paralyze the nerve centers and lessen our chances to locate the trouble. Dr. Chapman has very well said, "Pain is the cry of a hungry nerve for better blood supply." And we say, yes, for better weapons to fight for perfect circulation, despite the various obstructions along the nerve channel and nerve endings where pain can be traced and found with the slightest pressure. We may take a person in perfect health with a perfect circulatory system and find no pain whatever in spite of all the pressure you can possibly bring to bear on any part of the foot. You will meet a few really healthy individuals, but they are few and far between, for it seems that the majority of mankind have some form of an ailment.

ONE HEALTHY YOUNG MAN

I was invited to dinner one evening by a patient of mine whose son from Buffalo was to be present. His mother, Mrs. C., tried to impress me with the idea that she was greatly worried over his condition, the nature of which she would not reveal, but left me to find where the trouble might be. As I proceeded in the usual way, trying various reflexes, I found not the slightest tenderness anywhere. I did not wish to disappoint Mr. C. or myself by being unable to locate the trouble, so after a most thorough tryout I had to give up, and in a way holding my breath said, "You really must be in perfect health." At this remark I was soon relieved to see the whole family smile and assure me that this occasion had been planned as a test case to see if this method was correct. Only a week before Mr. C. had passed an examination for a twenty thousand dollar Life Insurance policy with the company's compliments on his unusually wonderful health.

It is interesting to encounter experiences similar to this. So often people think their feet are perfectly well, and will say to you, "Oh, my feet are the best part of me." The real fact is, their bodily ailments have not yet been realized, only in the form of an occasional headache, or perhaps some indigestion now and then, which nature has sent out in the form of a danger signal.

VARIOUS METHODS

Remember there are many successful methods of helping various ailments. The physician can often give a pill or write a prescription containing some herb extraction equalizing the acidity, or alkalinity of the blood stream. This increases the vitality of the body sufficiently to rid these nerve extremities of any obstruction caused by an acid formation, without the method outlined in this book. But it is an indisputable fact that we can help nature to perform her important duties more efficiently and obtain quicker and more lasting results along any line of practice by the addition of this simple method of massage herein outlined, which can be administered successfully by any nurse or attendant.

IMPORTANCE OF PROPER CIRCULATION

Every practitioner will admit the importance of proper circulation in order to have a body free from congestion and the hundred and one ailments caused from this condition. No one can deny the well known fact that circulation is life; stagnation is death. As long as any part of the one hundred percent normal circulation is being cut off from any one or more parts of the body, be it only that of a tiny gland, we begin to feel the effect in one way or another; with a pain here or an ache there. Nature tries to cry out and tell us these various defects in time to remedy them, but we pay no attention and try to silence the alarm with some deadening pill. But as a chain is no stronger than its weakest link, so our body is no stronger than its weakest point.

Now remember nature will do her part if we give her half a chance. So if we can learn some simple way to stimulate the normal circulation by relieving the congestion in the various nerve endings in the feet, is it not worth some careful consideration? I do not ask you to believe something that has not been already proven beyond any doubt; I only ask you to try it out for yourself, and watch for results.

A CONCLUDING THOUGHT

In concluding this work on "Stories The Feet Can Tell," let me remind you again that massage in any form is only a means of exercise, a means of equalizing the circulation.

We all know circulation is life. Stagnation is death. Everything around us that is alive is in motion.

Everything in the universe is governed by the law of motion, which is one of God's great infallible laws of nature. It is from the earth, sun, and water which are constantly in motion that we receive our creative forces which are followed by growth, maturity and decay. Nothing stands still. Our vitality is either increasing or decreasing according to the quality and circulation of our bloodstream.

Study for a moment the life of a sturdy oak, which from a tiny acorn grows. Stop and observe how it lifts its leafy arms toward Heaven to receive from the passing breezes the exercise necessary to strengthen its root supply, increasing the capacity to gather moisture and nourishment necessary to furnish and keep the sap flowing freely through every part. If we cut off the roots sufficiently to rob it of its life-giving sap, how long will the tree be green and full of life?

In the face of this shall we forget the necessity of keeping our whole body in motion; every part in perfect rhythm.

It is my sincere wish that this new technique of compression massage on the reflexes of the feet will stand side by side with other great therapy works in the onward march of science and progress.

EUNICE D. INGHAM

INDEX

INDEX

ILLUSTRATIONS

ILLUSTRATIONS

NOTES